Cannabis Medicine

What You Need to Know

By Ryder Management Inc

Epigraph

*"There were never so many able, active minds at work on the problems of disease as now, and all their discoveries are tending toward the simple truth that -> **you can't improve on nature.**"*
Thomas Edison in 1902

"Nature Heals: The Doctor's task consists in strengthening the natural healing powers, to direct them, and especially not to interfere with them."
Hippocrates

"The whole is greater than the sum of its parts"

Aristotle

Preface

Cannabis occupies one of the most important chapters in the history of world medicine. Abundantly supplied by nature, cannabis is non-toxic, safe and has a wide range of applications in treating human health and disease. For centuries, cannabis treated a number of mental health disorders as well as physical ailments and dysfunctions.

When did we become incapable of choosing what is best for ourselves? In other words, when did we give up the right to choose our own health care?

Over the past several decades, the federal government has sponsored research to find negative effects in cannabis, while blocking research into the positive effects. Ironically, however, in the government's quest to search for the harm in this plant, a remarkable amount of evidence appeared on the astounding medicinal benefits in this plant.

Cannabis, as a *drug* in its natural form, has four main advantages that make it unique as a therapeutic remedy:

Cannabis is the least toxic of all available drugs

Cannabis has a large range of therapeutic uses, none of which are toxic nor produce any side effects

Cannabis behaves in a way that is very different from synthetic drugs; and

Cannabis use is safe to use in combination with other drugs.

The distinction of a drug over an industrial variety of this plant occurred with the adoption of the Single Convention on Narcotic Drugs. The historical distinction was based on the plant's ratio of THC to CBD as determined by gas chromatography, a method that has revealed a number of faults.

The purpose of this book is to further the understanding of the medicinal benefits in cannabis, including the terpenes and other cannabinoids besides THC and CBD.

Contrary to conventional medicine's practice of dividing the body into its individual parts, the individual parts of a plant is greater than the sum of its parts in that the synergistic benefits it provides to the body as a whole, is far more effective than a synthetic part devised in a lab.

Table of Contents

Introduction

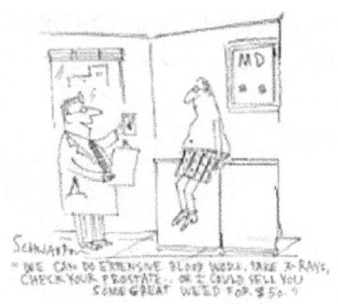

It is actually quite simple: the medical use of cannabis has roots dating back to pre-recorded history.

Cannabis is more than just the ratio of THC to CBD. Cannabis is far more complex than just these two commercialized cannabinoids -THC and CBD. Cannabinoids, terpenes and other secondary metabolites found in the cannabis plant elicit various medicinal and health effects in our body. These compounds bind to receptor sites in the cell walls of our body, proving an historical relationship to this plant.

The misinformation surrounding medical cannabis is astounding. This conflict creates an enormous amount of confusion for "medical marijuana" patients. This confusion is deliberate *and created by the champions of prohibitionists, whom continue to ignore the scientific facts of* medical cannabis, in its natural form.

In the early 20th century, cannabis regulation began with a group of laws and social policies, serving a variety of private ulterior motives, and born of the authoritarian notion that citizens are incapable of handling "mind-affecting" substances on their own, as responsible adults.

In the nineteenth century, the various forms of cannabis distillations, tinctures and elixirs were the third most favored type of medicine by both doctors and patients alike.

Throughout human history, cannabis and its derivatives have held a paramount position in day-to-day therapeutic practice. *Supplied in abundance by nature, cannabis is a non-toxic, safe and effective application for a number of maladies including 'neuralgia, gout, tetanus, hydrophobia, epidemic cholera, convulsions, chorea hysteria, mental depression, insanity, and uterine haemorrhage'.* G. Wood and F. Bache, Dispensatory of the United States (1854), p.339

Legacy of Medicinal Use

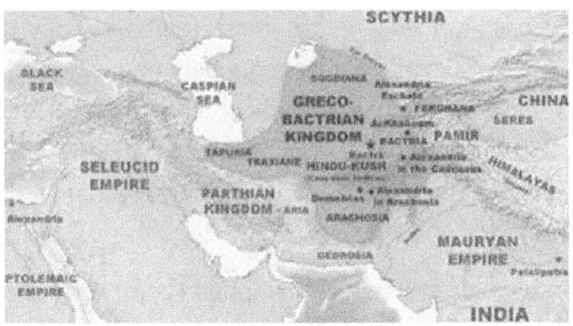

Ancient evidence reveals cannabis medicine dates back to pre-historic time.

The earliest known medical texts, whether they are **Sumerian or Assyrian cuneiform tablets**, **Mesopotamian clay tablets** (ancient Near East now modern day Iraq, Syria, and Kuwait), **Egyptian papyrus scrolls**, **Chinese tables**, **Atharva Veda** (an ancient Indian collection of sacred texts of unknown source), etc., all speak of the medicinal use of Cannabis in the **past tense**. In addition, none of the earliest recordings, in any ancient medical text, suggests discovering cannabis as medicine for the first time. These earliest texts, in keeping with their mandate, pass on a history of known medical remedies, of which cannabis is revered. In these ancient recordings on plant medicine, cannabis is most commonly described in the form of a tincture or a tea.

It is fascinating to learn that 789 grams of cannabis was discovered in a 2,700 year old excavated Gushi tomb located within the *Yanghai Tombs – Cemetery of Pastoral Nomads* in the *Turpan Oasis, Xinjiang Province of Northwestern China*. The *Yanghai Tombs* belong to the Subeixi Culture, a nomadic tribe prosperous over 3,000 years ago.

In addition to the above, in the *Caucasus Mountains of southern Russia*, archaeologists have confirmed that their excavation from a *2,400 year old Scythian burial* included sold gold bongs and substances that were later *confirmed to be opium and cannabis*.

There is consensus among experts of **Egyptian hieroglyphs** (writing system of the ancient Egyptians) that the Egyptian word for cannabis was 'smsm-t' – pronounced 'shemshemet'. The Ebers Papyrus, c. 1550 BC, is among Ancient Egypt's oldest and most important of their medical papyrus and it includes the use of medical cannabis in various preparations and for treating a range of disorders. However, some scholars believe that the Ebers Papyrus is a compilation of older works, dating as far back as 3400 BC.

British archaeologist Reginald Campbell Thompson (1876-1941) spent 50 years deciphering **19,000 Assyrian cuneiform tablets** recovered from an archaeological site in the ancient **Near East** ruins of Nineveh, across the Tigris River from the modern day **Iraqi** city of Mosul. **Assyria** was a major **Mesopotamian** East Semitic kingdom and empire of the **ancient Near East** and existed as an independent state from the 25th century BC to 605. (Wikipedia)

According to Thompson, cannabis was known as *'azallu'* in ancient Assyrian and out of the 19,000 clay tablets examined, 600 tablets related to *'Material Medica'* and contained citations to cannabis.

Historians have noted that George Washington grew hemp not only for fiber but also for medicinal use. Since Washington kept journals, in the 1967 book "The Book of Grass: An Anthology of Indian Hemp" by George Andrews, he argues about the much discussed August 7, 1765 entry in George Washington's journal:

August 7, 1765 "...began to separate the Male from the Female Hemp at ... rather too late."

Mentioning separating male from female is to prevent fertilization and to produce the medicinal benefits derived from female buds.

Despite the above, they say that William B. O'Shaughnessy, an Irish physician introduced cannabis into Western medicine in the 1840's (the Victorian era) after learning of its medicinal value while working in India for the British East Indies Company. Cannabis *medicine was promoted for analgesic, sedative, anti-inflammatory,* antispasmodic, and anticonvulsant properties.

Shortly after O'Shaughnessy published his findings, Cannabis made its first appearance into the 1851 and 3rd edition of the U.S. Pharmacopoeia. Every edition after the third, up to and including the 11th edition in 1936, would expand on the standardization and dosing of this medicine. In fact, the U.S.P. dictated the exact parts of the plants to use, the exact method of preparation and later, a standard for potency. Unfortunately, due to political pressure, Cannabis was removed from the 12th edition of the U.S.P. 1942. In the mid-1800's cannabis was known to successfully treat neuralgia, tetanus, typhus, cholera, rabies, dysentery, alcoholism, opiate addiction, anthrax, leprosy, incontinence, gout, convulsive disorders, tonsillitis, insanity, excessive menstrual bleeding and uterine bleeding, among others.

Early 20th century use of medical cannabis can also be found in the **1900** JAMA - *Journal of the American Medical Association* - one of the leading medical journals published in the United States. Within the 1900 version of this esteemed journal, **"Cannabis Indica"** was described as *"first stimulating, and later sedative"*. This authoritative publication further described **Cannabis Indica** as *"one of the best of anodynes in multiple neuritis"*; *"It is unequaled to quiet the neuroses (anxiety, depression)"*; *"...it is seen to provide evident improvement in diabetes ... and it is very useful in relieving intolerable itching and burning in all neuroses of the skin."* ***JAMA 1900, V.35, p 457***

According to the **1910** textbook *"Therapeutics, Materia Medica and Pharmacy"* by S.L.Potter, medical cannabis was recommended for over 45 specific diseases and ailments including, but not limited to: asthma, bladder infections, kidney disease (albuminuria), insomnia, pain, whooping cough (pertussis), pulmonary tuberculosis (phthisis), tetanus, urinary disorders, uterine cancer plus many more.

Classification by Government

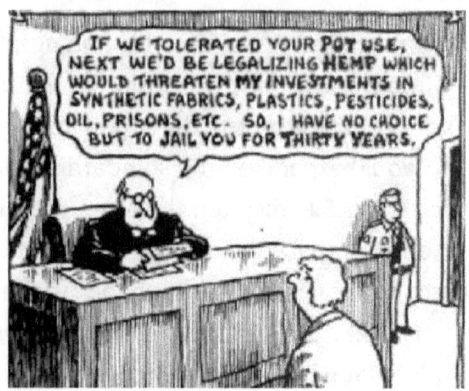

Whether the genus cannabis consists of one species (with various sub-species) or a genus that is polytypic, consisting of more than one species, is an ongoing debate.

In 1753, **Carolus Linnaeus** was familiar with European hemp that was widely cultivated at that time. He considered cannabis to be a single species and named his discovery Cannabis sativa L (L. indicating the authority who first named the species, in this case Linnaeus). The binomial nomenclature *"Cannabis sativa"* was published in the 1753 edition of *Linnaeus in Species Plantarum* in 1753, an internationally accepted publication still considered the starting point for modern botanical binomial nomenclature (system of names and rules for inclusion in any classification) of the day.

In 1785, **Jean-Baptiste de Lamarck** published his discovery of a second species obtained from India that he named *Cannabis indica Lam.* He described this second species as having poorer fiber quality than C. sativa but greater intoxicating qualities.

In 1924, **Dmitri E. Janischewsky**, a Russian botanist, identified a third type of cannabis growing wild in Central Russia. Named Cannabis ruderalis Janisch, this third species of cannabis differs from C. sativa and C, Indica in that C. Ruderalis flowers based on age rather than life cycle. Referred to as "autoflowering" C. ruderalis does not depend on the sun to reproduce, rather it reproduces based on age. As a ruderal plant, one that survives despite all odds, it is clear that cannabis has fought to be here.

In 1918, Dr. Andrew Wright, an agronomist and steward of the Wisconsin hemp industry, wrote, "There are three fairly distinct types of hemp: that grown for fiber, that for birdseed and oil, and that grown for drugs".

In 1971, with the adoption of the UN's Single Convention on Narcotic Drugs, the concentration of the most abundant cannabinoids in cannabis, namely THC and CBD, was analyzed both qualitatively (whether it is present) and quantitatively (how much there is). Chromatography, a method of separating like compounds in any given sample of organic matter, was considered the most objective in determining a plant's psychoactive activity.

Also in 1971, Fetterman et al, divided Cannabis plants into *two distinct chemical phenotypes* (chemotypes), **namely drug or fiber types**. According to this classification, if the ratio of THC to CBD is greater than one, the classification is automatically a 'drug chemotype'; otherwise, a ratio of less than one is a 'fiber chemotype'.

In 1973, Small and Beckstead identified **three distinct cannabis phenotypes** as follows

1. **Drug type** = THC/CBD > 1;

2. **Intermediate type** = THC/CBD close to one; and

3. **Fiber type** = THC/CBD < 1.

The above calculation is what today's government relies on today in determining drug identification.

Whether the genus Cannabis consists of one or more species has been widely debated (Small and Cronquist, 1976). Using gas chromatography in 1979 and following the work of Fetterman et al (1971), Canadian botanist Ernest Small and American taxonomist Arthur

Cronquist claimed to have differentiated indica strains from sativa strains based on their THC and CBD content.

Although CBD is promoted as the second most important cannabinoid after THC, evidence now exists that the results of early gas chromatography tests, tests used to classify cannabis strains into drugs or fiber, have been misinterpreted. The classification of a substance into drug or fiber chemotype was based on a ratio of THC to CBD as elucidated from gas chromatography, a method of separating like compounds in an organic sample. New information shows that the cannabinoid CBD was probably greatly over exaggerated due to the cannabinoid, CBC. Recently disclosed publicly, the cannabinoid *Cannabichromene or CBC* was **frequently misidentified as CBD or Cannabidiol** in the early use of gas chromatography as the method used to quantify THC and CBD content. The reason for this error is that CBC and CBD have the same retention times in gas chromatography results. (Russo et al, 2010)

Since the disclosure of the above limitation with gas chromatography along with the plethora of updated and current research on cannabis, governments continue to use the ratio of THC to CBD to determine whether a given substance is *drug, non-drug, or a fiber strain* of Cannabis. In addition, current cannabis literature continues to exaggerate the benefits of CBD to the exclusion of other beneficial cannabinoids and corresponding terpenes.

This book uses the common terms of Sativa, Indica, and Hybrid when describing various Cannabis strains. As a side note, a discussion of the fiber side of hemp strains is beyond the scope of this book.

Cannabis Taxonomy

DOMAIN Eukarya
KINGDOM Plantae
PHYLUM Magnoliophyta
CLASS Magnoliopsida
ORDER Rosales
FAMILY Cannabaceae
GENUS *Cannabis*

The scientific system of classification divides all living things into groups called taxa. Plants are included in the kingdom of ***Plantae.*** The *Plant Kingdom* is divided into two taxa: broyophytes and *vascular* plants. *Vascular* plants are divided into two subgroups: seedless and *seeded*. The **seeded plants** further divide into Gymnosperms and *Angiosperms* that further divide into *divisions*. All *division* names end in *'pyhta'*. The division name for flowering plants is called *Magnoliophyta*. *Angiosperms* (*Magnoliophyta* or broadleaf flowering plants) produce seeds through flowering. *Angiosperms* are divided into *two taxa:* monocots and *dicots*. After the dicot Class, the taxa for Cannabis in descending order include **Order, Family, Genus, and Species**.

Family names end in 'aceae' and cannabis belongs to the family ***Cannabaceae.***

Plant taxonomy is an old science that historically used physical characteristics, called gross morphology, to systematically separate plants into similar groups. Plant taxonomy is slowly being absorbed into the new science of ***systematics*** due to the development of more sophisticated techniques in laboratory chemical analysis. Systematics is based on evolutionary similarities such as chemical makeup and reproductive features.

Within the plant order Urticales, Stephan Endlicher, an Austrian botanist, created a separate family, the Cannabaceae Family, in 1837. Moved to the Urticaceae family (nettle family) in 1880 by Bentham and Hooker, Cannabis was again moved in 1889 by Engler and Prantl to the

Moraceae or fig family. Taxonomists today assign Cannabis to the Cannabaceae or Moraceae family.

Under the APG III system, 2009 (Angiosperm Phylogeny Group III system) of flowering plants, plants belonging to the old Urticales order, along with four other families, now belong to the order *Rosales*. Therefore, the current systematic classification of Cannabis is as follows:

Division: Magnoliophyta (Angiosperms)

Class: Dicotyledon (dicot for short) is a flowering plant that produces two seed leaves when the seed germinates. Dicots are also referred to as *Magnoliopsida*)

Subclass: Archichlamydeae (subclass of dicots in which the flowers do not produce petals; *this subclass is rarely used now)*

Order: *Rosales* (before molecular phlogenetics became an important part of plant taxonomy, this order was known as *Urticales)*

Family: Cannabaceae

Genus: Cannabis

Species: Cannabis sativa L; Cannabis indica Lam; and Cannabis ruderalis Janisch, more commonly known as Sativa, Indica, and Ruderalis, respectively

Cultivars or strains: Over 700 strains have been developed and cultivated using sativa, indica, or hybrid strains.

Anatomy of Cannabis

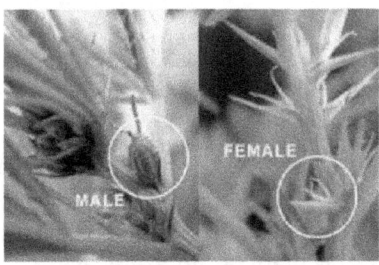

Cannabis is an annual plant since its life cycle completes within a single year. It is usually a dioecious plant, whereby the male and female reproductive organs develop on separate plants. The male plant produces *staminate* flowers (stamen) while the female plant produces *pistillate* flowers (pistils). The purpose of the male flower is to produce pollen to fertilize the female, whereas the purpose of the female flower is the production of achenes (seeds). If fertilization does not take place, the lack of seed formation induces the female plants to produce more flowers, leading to increased resin production with higher cannabinoid content.

The stamen on the male plant consists of a slender stalk called the filament that supports the oval shaped anthers - the part of the stamen that produces pollen. The sole function of the male cannabis plant is to pollinate the females.

The male cannabis plant will normally start to flower one to four weeks before the female and tends to grow straight up with the flowers developing in tight clusters near the top of the plant. Each male cannabis flower consists of five petal shaped *sepals*, which enclose or surround the sex organs. As each flower matures, the sepals open in a radiating pattern to reveal five pendulous anthers (usually referred to as stamens). Within the anthers, pollen is developed and these anthers ultimately split open, releasing pollen to the wind for transfer to awaiting pistillate female flowers. Mature anthers are described as resembling tiny bunches of bananas. Shortly after pollination takes place, the male plants wither and die allowing the female plants to flourish and produce a large quantity of seed for reproduction.

The female cannabis plant will generally start to flower when the average daily photoperiod is less than 12-13 hours per day. The female cannabis plant flowers later than the male. Once the female starts to flower, she will "fill out" as flowers develop from each leaf axil and growing tip. She will also stop growing in height.

The sex of a cannabis plants is anatomically visually indistinguishable until it starts flowering. However, molecular genetic markers have been found within the cannabis plant, which means that the plant's sex can be determined (with special testing equipment) before any visible signs are noticed.

After the male plant has finished shedding pollen, it dies and this event occurs before the seeds in the female plants ripen, usually four to eight weeks after fertilization.

The term 'Sinsemilla' (pronounced "seen-say-ME-yah") is from the Spanish word 'sin' = 'without' and 'semilla' meaning 'seed'; the Spanish word Sinsemilla therefore translates to mean 'without seeds' and relates to the unpollinated female flower of the cannabis plant. Although an alternate spelling is *sensimilla,* the misspelling probably results from phonetically sounding the word out.

Sinsemilla refers to the preferred cultivation technique rather than a generic strain. The production of sinsemilla requires the identification of both the female and male cannabis plants to ensure that the female plants are not pollinated.

Medicinal cannabis is specifically grown for the seedless inflorescence of the female cannabis plant. Inflorescence is the scientific name given to the cannabis bud.

Endocannabinoid System

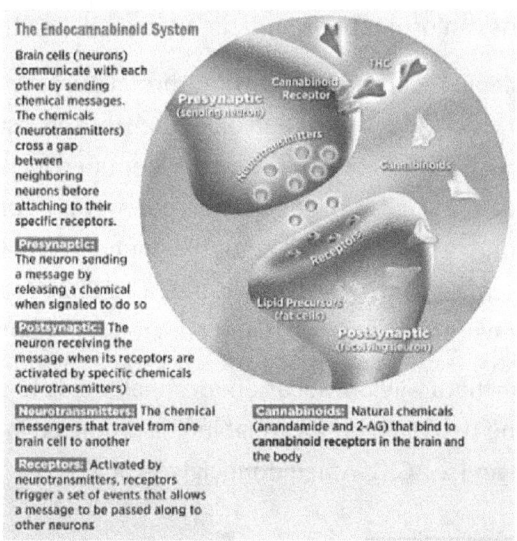

The Endocannabinoid System

Brain cells (neurons) communicate with each other by sending chemical messages. The chemicals (neurotransmitters) cross a gap between neighboring neurons before attaching to their specific receptors.

Presynaptic: The neuron sending a message by releasing a chemical when signaled to do so

Postsynaptic: The neuron receiving the message when its receptors are activated by specific chemicals (neurotransmitters)

Neurotransmitters: The chemical messengers that travel from one brain cell to another

Receptors: Activated by neurotransmitters, receptors trigger a set of events that allows a message to be passed along to other neurons

Cannabinoids: Natural chemicals (anandamide and 2-AG) that bind to cannabinoid receptors in the brain and the body

Perhaps the most important physiological system that establishes and maintains human health is our endogenous (located within the body) cannabinoid system - also known as the endocannabinoid system (ECS). Endocannabinoids and their cannabinoid receptors are located throughout our entire body, including our brain, organs, connective tissues, glands and immune cells. Although the endocannabinoid system performs different functions in each tissue, the overall objective of our ECS is that of homeostasis (to bring balance within the entire body).

The endocannabinoid system includes both the cannabinoid receptors and the endocannabinoids and they interact with each other in a way similar to that of "lock and key". The endocannabinoids are endogenous ligands produced by different body cells and act as perfect keys that join the cannabinoid receptors, which are cell membrane proteins that act as the lock. Phytocannabinoids act as missing keys, whenever the body is deficient in endocannabinoids, phytocannabinoids can help in this deficiency.

With its complex model of action in each of the immune system, body organs, and central nervous system, our endocannabinoid system is a bridge between body and mind. Understanding our endocannabinoid system might shed light on how states of consciousness can promote or impede our overall health.

Cannabinoid receptors are present throughout our entire body and thought to be more prevalent than any other receptor system found in our body. The two cannabinoid receptors identified include the CB1 receptor, found in our brain, central nervous system, connective tissue, glands, and organs; and the CB2 receptor, found in our stem cells, immune system and associated structures. The CB2 receptor was also recently discovered in our brain, liver, pancreas, and bone.

Our body naturally produces endocannabinoids to stimulate the CB receptors. The two main endocannabinoids produced in our body are anandamide and 2-AG (2-Arachidonoylglycerol).

Anandamide

Chemical formula: $C_{22}H_{37}NO_2$

First isolated in 1992, Anandamide, also known as - N-*Arachidonoylethanolamine or AEA*, is a neurotransmitter (chemical that enables cell communication) and endocannabinoid (produced within the body). The name Anandamide comes from the Sanskrit word ananda, meaning bliss, and the word amide, which refers to a type of acid in the body. Anandamide is widely known as the bliss compound. Research has found that yoga can increase this compound. In addition, a deficiency in anandamide has been linked to an increase in anxiety and stress.

An important role of **anandamide** is regulating appetite, pleasure, sleep patterns and pain. Anandamide also has an important role in balancing hormones and the reproductive system, however, more research is needed to further the understanding is this regard.

Anandamide has also been discovered in chocolate, somewhat explaining the blissful feeling while consuming it.

A report from NCIB shows that anandamide prevents the reproduction and spreading of cancer cells in breast cancer. This report also anandamide lowers ocular blood pressure.

Summary of anandamide's therapeutic uses: analgesic, pain reliever; angiogenic, causes blood vessels to split and form new blood cells; *anti-proliferative*, prevents cancer cell growth; *anxiolytic*, inhibits anxiety; *euphoriant*, promotes happiness and a sense of well-being; *neurogenic*, increases the growth of new brain cells in the area of the brain responsible for memory.

2-AG

Chemical formula: $C_{23}H_{38}O_4$

The other main endocannabinoid found in our body is known as 2-AG (2-Arachidonoylglycerol). 2-AG plays a complex and important role in various body processes including immunity and inflammation.

The endogenous cannabinoid 2-AG is found in the brain in addition to its periphery. In a 2014 publication entitled *"An endogenous cannabinoid (2-AG) is neuroprotective after brain injury"* researchers found neuroprotective properties in 2-AG after brain injury. 2-AG also reduces *"**blood brain barrier"*** permeability in brain trauma following a concussive hit in a football injury.

2-Arachidonoylglycerol is an endogenous agonist of the CB1and CB2 receptors. As an ester, it is synthesized on-demand from cell membranes *arachidonic acid derivatives* and glycerol to stimulate the cannabinoid receptors.

Endocannabinoids, found throughout our central nervous system (CNS), are essential modulators of neurotransmitters, also called synaptic transmitters. Endocannabinoids are part of the lock and key system found in our body and are analogs (similar in chemical structure) to phytocannabinoids, the cannabinoids found in cannabis.

2-AG is the most abundant endocannabinoid found in our body and similar to anandamide, 2-AG plays a major role in appetite regulation, immune system function, and pain-management. It also plays a significant role in the prevention of cancer cell proliferation.

Secondary Plant Metabolites

When Aristotle said, *"The whole is greater than the sum of its parts"* surely he was referring to the healing powers of the cannabis plant, or any other medicinal plant for that matter. The synergy effect of all the compounds found in the cannabis plant, work in harmony, and is what gives this plant its unique and powerful healing abilities.

Plants produce a vast and diverse assortment of organic compounds, the great majority of which do not appear to contribute directly to its growth, development, and reproductive functions and are thus referred to as secondary metabolites. These secondary plant metabolites are limited to certain taxonomic groups in the plant kingdom, of which Cannabaceae is one. Primary plant metabolites are found in all plants, as these organic compounds are considered essential for growth, development, and reproduction, in plants.

Secondary metabolites are found to play a major role in the adaption of plants to their environment, defense mechanisms, and the ability to thrive. The secondary metabolites found in the cannabis plant include cannabinoids, terpenes, flavonoids, stilbenoids, alkaloids, lignans, and phenolic amides; however, some of these classes of compounds also include primary metabolite activity. The distinction between primary and secondary metabolite is based not only on chemical structure but also on function.

A number of terpenes and flavonoids that are found in the cannabis plant are also found in other medicinal herbs. However, cannabinoids in cannabis are unique and specific to this plant and has not been elucidated in any other plant species, not even hop (Humulus lubulus), which is in the same family as cannabis (the *Cannabaceae* Family).

Secondary plant metabolite research is only beginning to evolve in the west, particularly with respect to their healing benefits and their role in medicine. Cannabinoids, terpenes and flavonoids have come under increased attention in the scientific and medical community due to their proven pharmacological actions.

Cannabinoids and terpenes share the same biosynthetic pathways; both compounds are biosynthesized in the glandular trichomes of the sugar leaves and flowers and are accumulated in large quantities in the exuded resin.

Nature is unique in its makeup and no matter how hard the scientific or pharmaceutical industry tries, it is impossible to synthetically reproduce or recreate the full medicinal activity of nature, in a lab.

Cannabinoids

As secondary metabolites, cannabinoids are defined as a group of naturally occurring *terpenophenolic* compounds and unique to the cannabis plant. One of the chief functions of secondary plant metabolites, such as cannabinoids, is achieving optimal health to thrive. Other secondary plant metabolites found in the cannabis plant include terpenes, flavonoids, stilbenoids, alkaloids, lignans, and phenolic amides.

Cannabinoids are produced in the glandular trichomes (trichome cells) through a process known as biosynthesis, a process in which enzymes cause a series of chemical reactions to produce a more complex set of molecules out of smaller and simpler molecules.

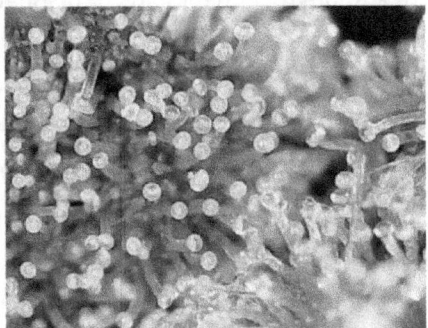

Magnified Glandular Trichomes

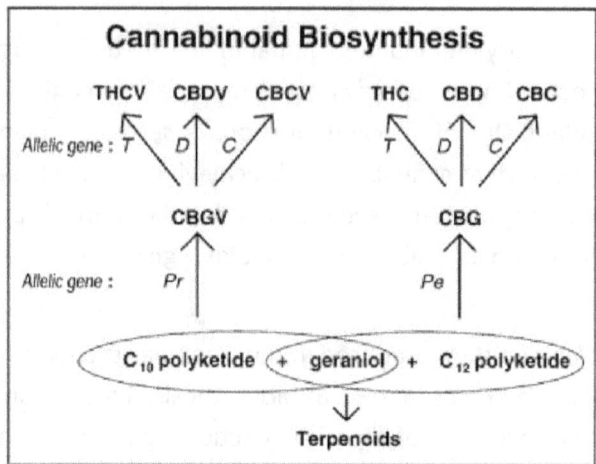

Cannabinoids (a.k.a. phytocannabinoids to distinguish them from those made in a lab called synthetic cannabinoids), have been divided into two main groups depending on their *"alkyl side chain"*: side chains, also called "tails", with three carbon atoms are called **propyl** side chains while those with five carbon atoms are known as **pentyl** side chains.

Cannabinoids that possess tails of five carbon atoms are defined as ***pentyl cannabinoids*** and are the most prevalent. The precursor to pentyl cannabinoids comes from ***olivetolic acid***. CBGA is the first biogenic cannabinoid formed in the cannabis plant from *olivetolic acid*. Other cannabinoids in the CBG group includes the 'propyl side chain analogs' (from the precursor CBGVA) and a monomethyl ether derivative (ex. CBGM).

The precursor to propyl cannabinoids comes from divarinic acid and forms ***Cannabigerivarinic acid or CBGVA*** as the first biogenic cannabinoid. Plants that develop divarinic acid originate from southern Africa, Afghan, and Pakistan (known as Indica strains). Distinguished from the *pentyl cannabinoids* with five chain tails, this group's tail consist of only three carbon atoms and is what defines them as ***propyl*** cannabinoids. The suffix used for *propyl* side chains is ***"varin"*** and these cannabinoids have specific medicinal benefits separate from the *'pentyl'* group of cannabinoids.

An example of the difference between the five chain tails and three chain tails is as follows: the chemical formula for Cannabigerolic acid (CBGA) is based on the chemical formula C_5H_{11} whereas the chemical formula that Cannabigerivarinic acid (CBGVA) is based on is C_3H_7.

The importance of this distinction is in the commercialization of cannabis as medicine. As previously mentioned, government control over this plant has emphasized the plant's THC to CBD ratio as the 'be-all-to-end-all' in terms of the knowledge over this plant. However, although the CBD cannabinoid can only be extracted from the cannabis seedless bud,, unless specifically bred for a high CBD content, CBD is actually found in very low doses, relative to the other cannabinoids. However, in order to treat childhood epilepsy, a medical cannabis strain was specifically bred for a large concentration of CBD. This strain was developed by the Stanley brothers in Colorado and was named Charlotte's Web, the little girl for whom it was successfully developed.

Synthesized from Olivetolic Acid (5 Carbon Tail)

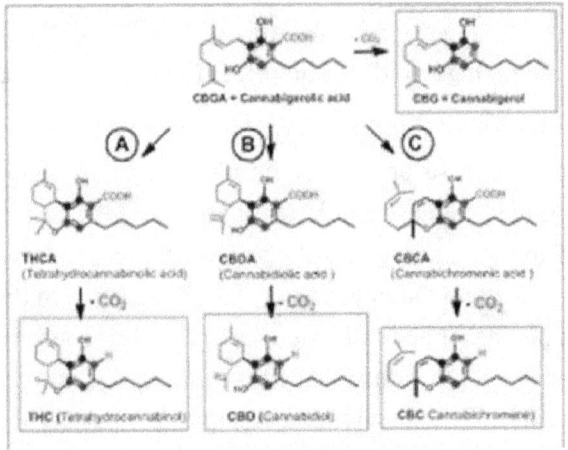

CBGA: Cannabigerolic acid – antibiotic, analgesic, anti-inflammatory

CBG: Cannabigerol – antibiotic, antibacterial, anti-cancer, antidepressant, antifungal, anti-inflammatory, analgesic, bone-stimulant

CBGAM: Cannabigerolic acid monomethyiether

CBGM: Cannabigerol monomethyiether

THCA: Tetrahydrocannabinolic acid – anticancer, anti-inflammatory, anti-spasmodic, antiproliferative, neuroprotective

THC: Tetrahydrocannabinol – euphoriant, analgesic, antimicrobial, anti-spasmodic, anti-inflammatory, antioxidant, antiemetic, appetite stimulant, neuroprotective, bronchodilator

CBDA: Cannabidiolic acid – anticancer, anti-inflammatory

CBD: Cannabidiol: analgesic, anti-epileptic, anti-inflammatory, anti-tumor, and more

CBT: Cannabitriol- a degraded form of CBD

CBDM: Cannabidiol monomethylether

CBCA: Cannabichromenic acid – antifungal, anti-inflammatory

CBC: Cannabichromene- analgesic, antimicrobial, antidepressant, anti-inflammatory, anti-insomnia, anti-prolific, bone and brain stimulant

CBCN: Cannabichromanon -

CBNA: Cannabinolic acid – Anti-inflammatory

CBN: Cannabinol – a degraded from of THC; sedative, analgesic, antibacterial, antibiotic; anticonvulsant; anti-inflammatory

CBND: Cannabinodiol

CBNM: Cannabinol methylether

CBLA: Cannabicyclolic acid – anti-inflammatory

CBL: Cannabicyclol – thought to be a heat generated artifact from CBC, in other words, a degraded form of CBC, it arises by exposure of CBC to UV radiation

CBEA: Cannabielsoic acid

CBE: Cannabielsoin – a metabolite of CBD

CBF: Cannabifuran

Synthesized from Divarinic Acid (3 carbon tail)

biogenetic pathway for cannabinoids with C3 side-chain.

CBGVA: Cannabigerovarinic acid – anti-inflammatory

CBGV: Cannabigerovarin

THCVA: Tetrahydrocannabivarinic acid – anti-inflammatory, neuroprotective

THCV: Tetrahydrocannabivarin – Antiepileptic, anti-convulsive, bone stimulant, analgesic, euphoriant, anorectic (appetite suppressant), bone stimulant

CBNV: Cannabinovarin – bone stimulant

CBDVA: Cannabidivarinic acid – anti-inflammatory

CBDV: Cannabidivarin – non-psychoactive, anti-convulsive, bone stimulant

CBCVA: Cannabichromivarinic acid - anti-inflammatory

CBCV: Cannabichromivarin

CNLV: Cannabicyclovarin

CBTV: Cannabitriolvarin

CBTVE: Ethoxy-cannabitriolvarin

CBV: Cannabivarin

CBVD: Cannabinodivarin

CBG

Analgesic	Borneol, Myrcene
Anti-bacterial	α-Pinene, β-Caryophyllene, Cineol, Humulene, Limonene, Linalool, Terpinolene
Anti-cancer	β-Caryophyllene, Citronellol, Humulene, Limonene, Myrcene
Anti-depressant	Cineol, Limonene, Linalool
Anti-fungal	α-Pinene, β-Caryophyllene, Caryophyllene oxide, Limonene, Nerlidol, Terpinolene
Bone Stimulant	

Although first discovered in 1964 as a constituent in hash, it was not until 1975 that scientists discovered that the precursor to all cannabinoids was in fact, *Cannabigerolic acid (CBGA)*. This discovery contrasted the previous literature claiming that CBD was the precursor to THC.

Cannabigerol (CBG) plays the primary role in the overall effects of cannabis and works behind the scene providing most of the medical effects of cannabis. CBGA and CBGVA are the precursors to THCA, CBCA, CBDA and THCVA, CBCVA, CBDVA respectively. When these cannabinoids are activated through decarboxylation, each lose their A atom.

CBGA is formed in the cannabis plant when *geranyl pyrophosphate* combines with *olivetolic acid*. On the other hand, **CBGVA** is formed in the cannabis plant when a derivative of *olivetolic acid*, called *divarinolic acid* binds with the substrate *geranyl pyrophosphate*. CBGVA is able to *cyclize*, just like CBGA, and form three more cannabinoids (CBCVA, THCVA, and CBDVA).

When these raw or acid cannabinoids are activated through heat, a process known as decarboxylation (decarb, for short) a carbon atom from the carbon chain is removed, producing the active cannabinoids CBCV, THCV and CBDV, of which, **THCV** has been shown to have very beneficial healing properties. The reverse process of decarboxylation is called carboxylation, which is the first chemical step in what is known as photosynthesis (the addition of CO_2 to a compound).

CBG is said to be limited to specific strains, relative to THC and CBD. However, in analyzing the footprint of numerous strains, CBG is found to be higher than CBD in most strains unless the strain is bred specifically for a high CBD content.

The Cannabigerol group of cannabinoids consists of six CBG type cannabinoids including CBGA – Cannabigerolic acid, CBG - Cannabigerol, CBGVA – Cannabigerovarinic acid, CBGV - Cannabigerovarin, CBGAM – Cannabigerolic acid monomethyiether, and CBGM – Cannabigerol monomethylether.

Cannabigerol is non psychoactive and has been shown to stimulate the growth of new brain cells, including in the elderly. CBG also stimulates bone growth, is antibacterial, anti-tumor, and helps combat insomnia.

Although the media and emerging commercial industry report the benefits of only THC and CBD, a number of patent applications have been filed for a number of specific diseases using cannabigerol and cannabigerol like compounds as an effective remedy. These patents cite cannabigerol and/or cannabigerol like compounds for the treatment of pain, cancer, neurodegenerative disease, brain injury or damage, acquired brain injury, age related inflammatory and more.

THC – Tetrahydrocannabinol

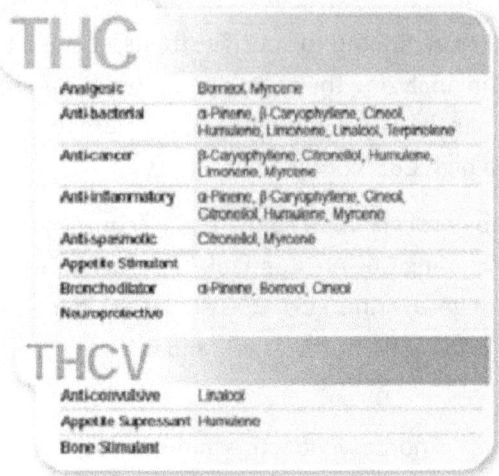

Although THC was first isolated in 1942, its correct structure did not properly take place until 1964 when it was elucidated by Dr. Raphael Mechoulam of Israel.

THC is the group of cannabinoids that are associated with the 'high'. THC has been found to be beneficial since THC mimics the action of anandamide, the neurotransmitter produced naturally in your body and which binds with the cannabinoid receptors in the brain.

Contrary to popular belief, THC has a number of positive effects on brain cells. THC is considered a "neuroprotectant" since it is able to protect brain cells from damage caused by inflammation and oxidative stress. In addition, scientists have shown how THC can even promote the growth of new brain cells through the process of neurogenesis. Dr. Xia Zhang of the University of Saskatchewan stated, "Most drugs of abuse suppress neurogenesis. Cannabis, on the other hand, promotes neurogenesis."

THC is a bronchial dilator, which means, similar to a cough drop; THC opens up your lungs to help clear them of smoke and dirt. Nicotine does the complete opposite in that it makes your lungs bunch up making it harder to clear your lungs by coughing.

THC cannabinoids possess a high UV-B absorption affinity.

In small moderate doses, THC promotes tranquility and a light sleep that includes pleasurable dreams followed by an easy awakening.

A summary of the beneficial effects of THC include *analgesic*, muscle relaxant and antispasmodic; *bronchodilator*; neuroprotective antioxidant; antipruritic agent in cholestatic jaundice, and it has 20 times the anti-inflammatory ability to that of aspirin along with twice its hydrocortisone.

THCV – Tetrahydrocannabivarin

THCV or Tetrahydrocannabivarin is the propyl form of THC. THCV is said to be strongly psychoactive, inducing a euphoric high. THCV is said to be more strongly psychoactive than THC, the duration of its effects are shorter, sometimes by as much as one half.

Recently THCV, alongside CB1 receptor antagonists, showed potential to combat diseases such as epilepsy.

THCV acts to simultaneously block the CB1 receptor and activate the CB2 receptor, which is very important in the treatment of liver disease and inflammation-associated obesity.

The medicinal effect of THCV include anticonvulsive and anti-epileptic since it is able to reduce convulsions and seizures; able to counter anxiety, stress, and panic disorders without suppressing emotions; controls panic associated with the Fight or Flight response; reduces tremors associated with Alzheimer's, Parkinson's as well as other neurological disorders. THCV is also considered an anorectic in that it diminishes appetite and consequently, assists with weight loss. It is also has analgesic, anti-inflammatory and bone stimulant properties and has excellent potential in treating osteoporosis and similar ailments.

CBN – Cannabinol

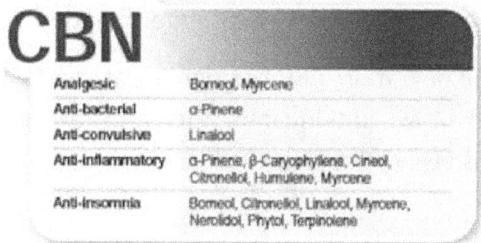

CBN	
Analgesic	Borneol, Myrcene
Anti-bacterial	a-Pinene
Anti-convulsive	Linalool
Anti-inflammatory	a-Pinene, β-Caryophyllene, Cineol, Citronellol, Humulene, Myrcene
Anti-insomnia	Borneol, Citronellol, Linalool, Myrcene, Nerolidol, Phytol, Terpinolene

In **1898**, CBN or Cannabinol was the first significant compound isolated from Cannabis sativa L. by Dunstan and Henry. (Levine, 1944) In Joseph Levine's 1944 communication 'Origin of Cannabinol', he writes, *"The purpose of this present communication is to report the formation of Cannabinol through the spontaneous degradation of tetrahydrocannabinol ..."*

CBN was also the first cannabinoid to be isolated from a red oil extract of cannabis at the end of the 19th century. Its structure was elucidated in the early 1930's by R.S. Cahn and its chemical synthesis first achieved in the laboratories of Roger Adams in the US and Lord Todd in the UK.

Cannabinol or CBN is the primary product of THC degration. There is very little of this cannabinoid in a fresh cured harvest since it usually occurs through aging from improper preservation techniques for THC. The presence of this cannabinoid increases in proportion to the decrease of THC content. The presence and quantity of CBN is a good indication of the age or improper treatment of your cannabis.

CBN is not directly produced through the plant's metabolism; rather, it is formed from degration of THC during drying, storing, or excessive heat. In fact, since CBN does not exist in freshly and carefully dried cannabis, if it is present, it is a good indication that the product was incorrectly handled.

THC degrades more rapidly during the first year after harvest relative to subsequent years. It has been suggested that the age of cannabis can be determined by looking at the THC to CBN ratio; however, since this ratio was used to classify drug from fabric variety, the THC to CBD ratio is irrelevant in this determination.

Regardless of degration, CBN has significant analgesic, anti-bacterial, anticonvulsive, anti-inflammatory, and anti-insomnia properties. CBN is also the strongest cannabinoid for promoting sleep.

CBD – Cannabidiol

CBD	
Analgesic	Borneol, Myrcene
Anti-anxiety	Linalool, Limonene
Anti-bacterial	α-Pinene, β-Caryophyllene, Cineol, Humulene, Limonene, Linalool, Terpinolene
Anti-cancer	β-Caryophyllene, Citronellol, Humulene, Limonene, Myrcene
Anti-convulsive	Linalool
Anti-depressant	Cineol, Limonene, Linalool
Anti-emetic	
Anti-inflammatory	α-Pinene, β-Caryophyllene, Cineol, Citronellol, Humulene, Myrcene
Anti-insomnia	Borneol, Citronellol, Linalool, Myrcene, Nerolidol, Phytol, Terpinolene
Anti-ischemic	Caryophyllene oxide
Anti-psychotic	
Anti-spasmotic	Citronellol, Myrcene
Bone Stimulant	
Immunosuppresive	
Neuroprotective	

CBDV	
Anti-convulsive	Linalool
Bone Stimulant	

Cannabidiol (CBD) is said to be the second most studied cannabinoid and was the second cannabinoid after CBN to be discovered. Cannabidiol was first isolated in 1940 by Roger Adams and colleagues in the US; however, it was not until 1963 that its proper structure was elucidated by Mechoulam and Shiva.

Cannabidiol is the most highly studied cannabinoid after THC. In contrast to THC, CBD has a relatively low affinity for the CB1 receptor, indicating that many of its pharmacologic properties are CB1 independent.

Contrary to most publications, a large majority of cannabis strains contain very little CBD, unless they are specifically bred to contain a larger quantity.

Cannabidiol is non-psychoactive and is effective in treating skin-disorders, drug addiction, epilepsy, obsessive-compulsive behavior, cancer, Alzheimer's disease, liver disease, heart disease, improves brain function, and more. CBD also contains universal anti-inflammatory properties.

CBC – Cannabichromene

CBC	
Analgesic	Borneol, Myrcene
Anti-bacterial	α-Pinene, β-Caryophyllene, Cineol, Humulene, Limonene, Linalool, Terpinolene
Anti-cancer	β-Caryophyllene, Citronellol, Humulene, Limonene, Myrcene
Anti-depressant	Cineol, Limonene, Linalool
Anti-fungal	α-Pinene, β-Caryophyllene, Caryophyllene oxide, Limonene, Nerlidol, Terpinolene
Anti-inflammatory	α-Pinene, β-Caryophyllene, Cineol, Citronellol, Humulene, Myrcene
Anti-insomnia	Borneol, Citronellol, Linalool, Myrcene, Nerolidol, Phytol, Terpinolene
Bone Stimulant	

The pentyl (C5) side chain of cannabichromene (CBC) was first identified in 1966 by Claussen et al, Gaoni, and Mechoulam

Both the pentyl and propyl (3 carbon side chain) groups of cannabichromene acids (CBCA and CBCVA) were described as racemic (no visual activity) in early research, due mainly to the difficulty with which scientists had describing its mechanism of action in isolated terms.

Cannabichromene has now been found to be 10 times more effective in treating anxiety and stress relative to *Cannabidiol (CBD).* GW Pharma has filed a patent application for their invention of using CBC in a medicament for treating depression and other mood disorders. CBC is the third most abundant cannabinoid, quantitatively, found in cannabis.

CBC is structurally similar to the other main natural (phyto) cannabinoids and is actually the second most abundant cannabinoid found in cannabis, despite CBD receiving all the attention in this regard. Although CBD was promoted as the second most important cannabinoid found in the cannabis plant, recent evidence shows that those early gas chromatography separation techniques employed, greatly over exaggerated CBC as CBD. In the mid-seventies, it was discovered that CBC was frequently misidentified as CBD using gas chromatography as a separation technique, because CBC and CBD have the same retention times when gas chromatography is used. (**Russo et al, 2010**)

Current research shows that CBC provides pain relief through its interaction with THC. It is now proven that CBC increases the pain relieving ability of THC in a synergistic way, one that is not achievable if CBC or THC acts alone.

CBC also inhibits inflammation and helps the body establish homeostasis. In addition, CBC stimulates bone growth and has strong anti-proliferative effects in that it inhibits the growth of cancer tumors. In addition, CBC has anti-depressant effects that are as much as 10 times greater than that of CBD. Studies also show that CBC has demonstrated sedative properties that promote relaxation.

Italian researchers made waves with a 2013 study, which suggests CBC, together with CBD, and cannabigerol (CBG), supports brain growth in adults.

In 1982, the University of Mississippi published a study showing CBC's strong anti-bacterial effects AND anti-fungal properties that is effective against Candida albicans.

All studies conclude that, like cannabis itself, CBC is not perfectly understood; studies do show that CBC has the highest medicinal use when used synergistically with other cannabinoids.

Cannabichromene or CBC has sedative effects, by itself, its analgesic (pain) effects are low; however, the analgesic effects increase when used in combination with THC, as gleaned from a sample on mice.

Recent research shows that CBC reduces edema swelling as well as inflammation of the intestinal tract. What sets this research apart is that CBC is able to fight inflammation without activating any known cannabinoid receptors. This might explain the synergy effects of CBC, since it does enhance the healing abilities of other cannabinoids.

Therapeutic uses include *analgesic*-pain reliever; *antibacterial*-inhibits bacterial growth; *anti-inflammatory*-systemically reduces inflammation; *anti-prolific*-inhibits cancer cell growth; *anti-fungal*-inhibits the growth of fungus; *anti-depressant*-alleviates depression; *anti-insomnia*-improves sleep behavior; *bone stimulant*-promotes bone growth.

Hemp Oil Misbranded as CBD Oil

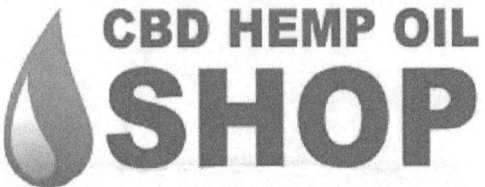

The *Hemp Industries Association* (**HIA**) is a North American non-profit association of the hemp trade. The HIA issued an official statement regarding the misbranding of hemp oil as "CBD Oil". The official statement emphasizes the need for accurate language in the marketplace to prevent consumers from being misled. *http://www.thehia.org/Resources/PressReleases/HIA-position-CBD-FINAL.pdf*

Medicinal cannabis plants with high CBD content may well contain less than 0.3% THC in their flowering tops and as such, are classified as "fiber" or "chemotype III" under the government's THC to CBD classification for determining drug type of a cannabis substance. To that end, medicinal cannabis strains bred for high CBD cannabinoid content are actually then classified as fiber strains under 'Section 7606 of the 2014 US Federal Farm Bill'.

It is important that you understand the difference between what is actually **CBD oil**, extracted from a medicinal cannabis plant bred for high CBD content and what is **hemp seed oil** (commonly known as hemp oil). Hemp seed oil is a much-needed dietary supplement. In contrast, essential oil extracted from medicinal cannabis, bred for a high CBD content, is, as you can see, a different story. Cannabidiol extracted from the bud of a medicinal cannabis plant bred for high CBD, is medicine.

The cannabinoid 'CBD' is not a component of hemp seed and as such, any labelling to that effect is misleading and assumed motivated by a desire to take advantage of the public and the grey area of the classification of CBD under Federal Law.

Hemp seed oil only contains about 25 parts per million (ppm) of CBD. In contrast, medicinal cannabis CBD oil, extracted from a medicinal strain bred for the cannabinoid CBD content, contains at least 150,000 ppm (parts per million) of this CBD cannabinoid. According to HIA official statement, *"It is important to be aware that most CBD purported to be in products mislabeled as 'hemp oil', is actually a by-product of large-scale hemp stalk and fiber-processing facilities in Europe where the fiber is the primary material produced at a large scale. CBD is not a product or component of hemp seeds, and any labelling to that effect is misleading and motivated by the desire to take advantage of the legal gray area of CBD under Federal Law."* They further state that hemp cultivars available to American farmers are not suitable for producing CBD.

Remember: Knowledge is Power!

Sativa versus Indica

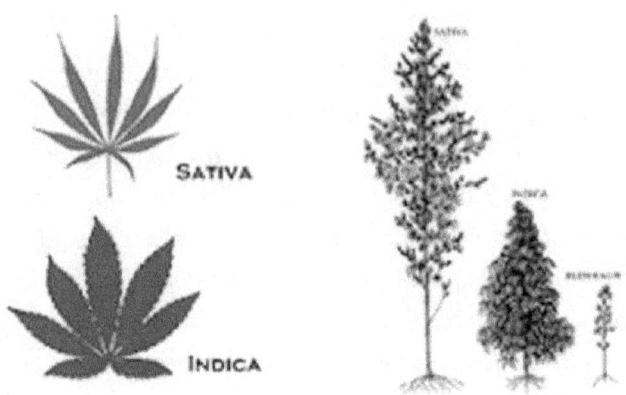

Understanding cannabis strains begins with an understanding of the broad categories from which the strain descends. The two most dominant species of cannabis plants are Sativa and Indica. Cross breeding of these species have produced a large number of hybrid strains each with their own unique characteristics. Since most medicinal cannabis strains are hybrids, the common accepted description of cannabis is whether the hybrid is Sativa dominant, Indica dominant or both (in which case, it is simply referred to as a hybrid). In the west, categorizing a plant as Indica or Sativa has created a number of debates over the years.

Geographic origin is a theory proposed for the Sativa-Indica classification. This theory purports that Sativa plants originate north of the 39th parallel whereas Indica plants originate south of the 39th parallel.

A prevalent classification system used by government authorities and the academic community alike focuses on a ***primary taxonomic criteria*** of cannabinoid composition. This system uses a ratio between the composition of THC and CBD quantity only. Historically, indica species had a high **THC: CBD ratio** (*drug type*) whereas Sativa plants had a high **CBD to THC ratio** (*referred to as fiber type*). Current literature indicates that Indica plants have a lower THC and higher CBD ratio relative to Sativa. Although still used today, this flawed system of classifying cannabis ignores the other cannabinoids and terpenes and the fact that cannabinoid composition fluctuates many times in a 24-hour period. In addition, since this system focuses only on a plants intoxicating ability as the prelude to species determination, it ignores distinctive **morphological** forms.

Morphology is the practice of classifying plants according to *physical appearance, characteristics and traits* and is applicable for describing the physical characteristics of the plant, but is not a hard and fast rule for determining the effects of the medicine. Under this classification, Indica plants are short and stout. Its leaves, relative to Sativa, are also shorter, wider and are a darker green. Indica leaves can also have a purple hue in their leaves whereas Sativa does not. Sativa plants grow tall and lanky and produce longer leaves with long thin leaf fingers. The leaf color of Sativa is a lighter shade of green relative to Indica.

The **effects** of Sativa and indica differ and are commonly distinguished as follows:

Sativa: uplifting and energetic; best suited for daytime use;

Indica: relaxing and calming; more of a body buzz; best suited for nighttime use

Despite the above classifications, breeders blur the morphology distinction between Sativa and Indica due to the mass hybridization of creating strains with a higher quantity of THC, larger yield and shorter flowering time.

The effects of individual cannabinoids are the same, regardless of whether it is Indica or Sativa, the synergy effects of the other cannabinoids and terpenes play a major role in the plant's medicinal effect.

Footprints of Cannabis Strains

In organic chemistry, the footprint of a cannabis plant is the amount of cannabinoids and terpenes present in a strain.

Cannabis has undergone major morphological and chemical changes over the past several decades. Selective breeding to meet the changing needs of the populace is the main reason for this change. The distinction between Sativa and Indica is now blurred and an argument is that strains today are no longer distinguishable between sativa and indica.

The massive hybridization of cannabis has led to a high level of homogeneity across strains. As breeders strived to increase potency and reduce the flowering time, virtually all strains have developed similar cannabinoid profiles; a relatively high level of THC, trace amounts of CBD and varying quantities of CBG, CBC and THCV. The main difference between popular strains these days are the result of variations in the terpene profiles.

In addition to modulating the effects of certain cannabinoids, terpenes also possess a number of medicinal effects on their own.

Cannatonic

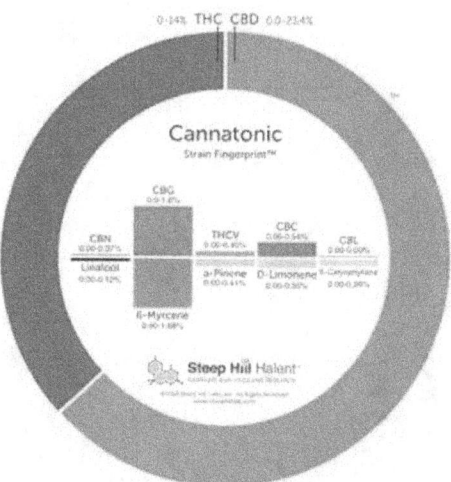

ACDC

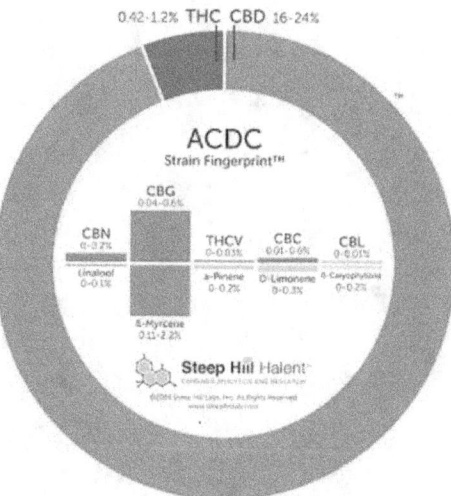

Harlequin

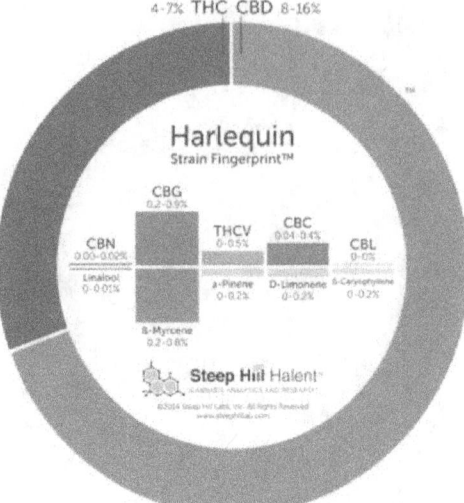

Girl Scout Cookies

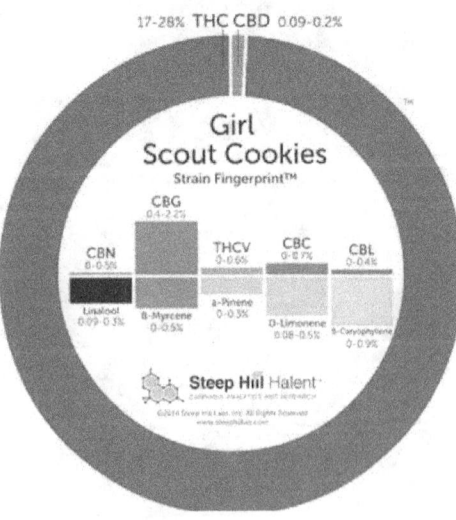

OG Kush

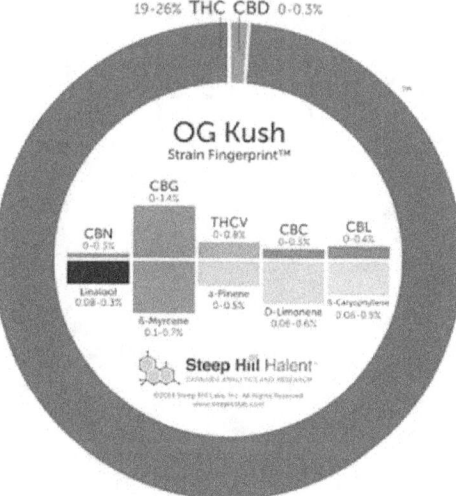

Durban Poison

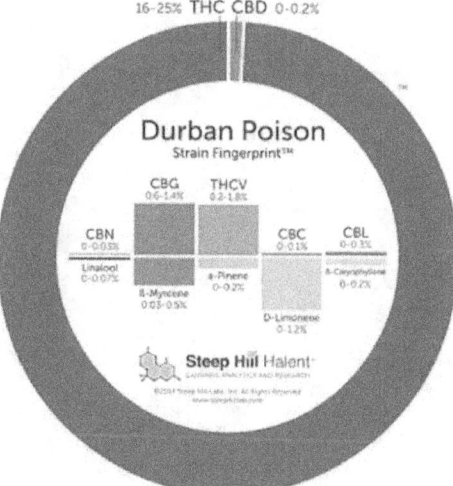

Trainwreck

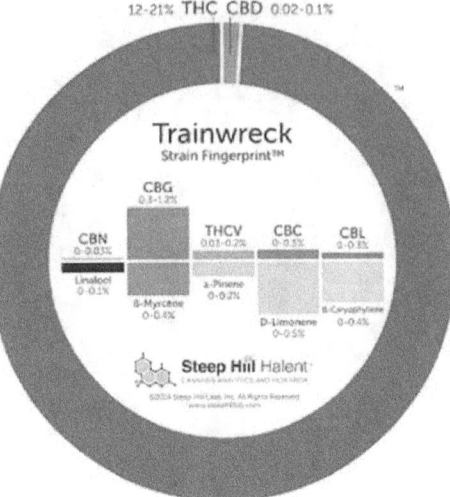

Sour Diesel

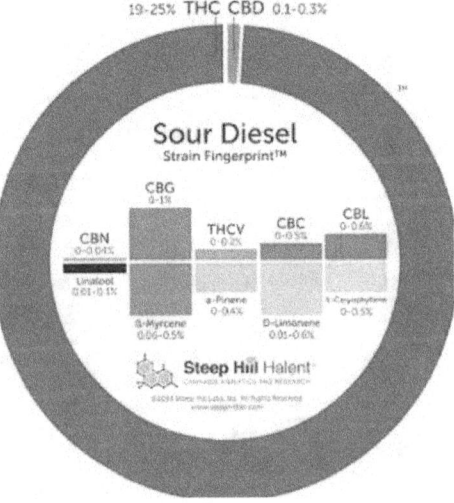

Chemdawg

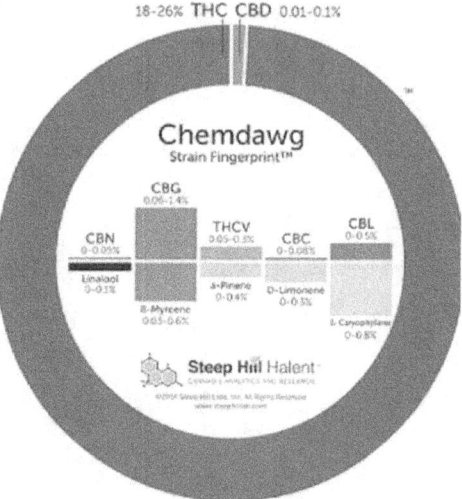

Green Crack

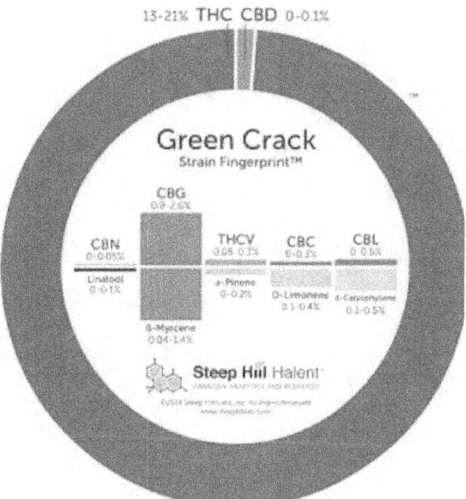

Agent Orange

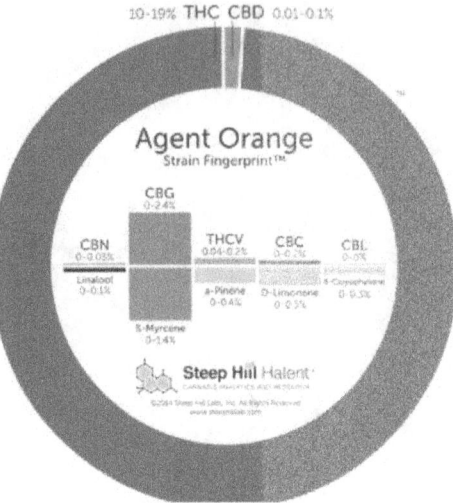

Jack Herer

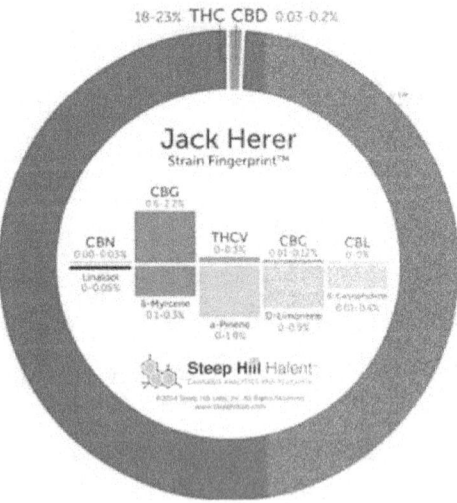

LA Confidential

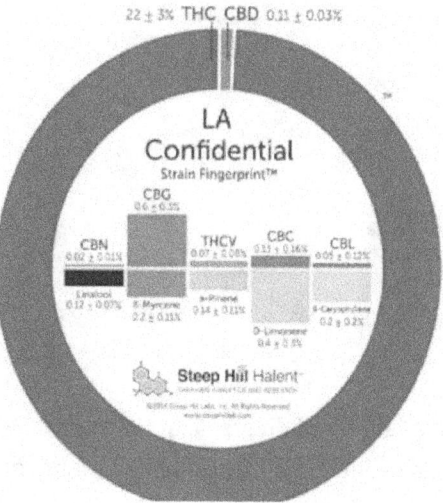

Terpenes

Name	Chemical Structure	Type
Myrcene		Acyclic
p-Menthane		Monocyclic
α-Pinene		Bicyclic

Terpenes are a large and diverse class of naturally occurring organic compounds produced by a number of plants of which many are "aromatic hydrocarbons" (sometimes called arenes). **Terpenes are produced in the same glandular trichomes that produce cannabinoids** and terpenes work synergistically with cannabinoids in their ability to heal. Examples of plants that contain terpenes include vegetables, fruit, herbs, spices, and botanicals such as roses. The name terpene comes from turpentine, which, in its raw form, is the sap from the Pine tree and which is terpene based.

Terpenes are important building blocks for certain essential odors, hormones, vitamins, steroids, resins, and cannabinoids.

Terpenes are very volatile, can evaporate quite easily and readily at normal temperatures, and are even liable to change rapidly and often unpredictably, sometimes for the worse. They are the compounds in cannabis, as with other plants, that give rise to the plant's unique scent.

When terpenes are chemically modified such as by oxidation, they are then referred to as terpenoids. Terpenoids are also known as isoprenoids. Terpenes and terpenoids are the primary constituents of the essential oils of many plants and flowers and are used quite extensively in aromatherapy, another form of 'alternative' healing.

Terpenes have a wide variety of medicinal benefits and each terpene contain a number of different properties that overlap with other terpenes and secondary metabolites, such as cannabinoids. When choosing a strain for your particular health needs, it is important to consider which terpenes are present in a particular strain, in addition to the cannabinoids.

Multiple studies give terpenes credit for their anxiolytic (anti-anxiety) and neuroprotector effects. Their capacity to modulate the effects of cannabinoids has been extensively studied and this fact is now quite well known in the scientific communities.

Although roughly 200 known and distinct terpenes have been identified in the cannabis plant, their relative concentration varies considerably among the many strains.

The most abundant terpenes in the Cannabis plant are the *monoterpenes* (molecular formula is $C_{10}H_{16}$) such as myrcene, pinene, limonene, linalool, and eucalyptol and the *sesquiterpene* (molecular formula is $C_{15}H_{24}$) caryophyllene. The variation in quantity of these terpenes is what causes the wide range of aromas in the various cannabis strains. Terpenes take part in the varied pharmacologic effects in cannabis **and produce synergy with the cannabinoids** (this fact will be repeated to stress its importance).

In the plant itself, the two main functions that terpenes have are protecting the plant against insects and herbivores as well as protecting it against high temperatures. *Monoterpenes* are more volatile and dominate in inflorescences (the cannabis buds) to repel insects. *Sesquiterpenes* are bitterer and more abundant on leaves as a way to protect the plant against herbivores.

As plants sense a rise in temperatures, they begin synthesizing more terpenes and release them when the temperature gets hot, regardless of whether it is day or night. At high temperatures, the terpenes evaporate which produce an airflow that cools the plant, lessening the loss of water vapor off its surface. The terpenes also cause the stickiness in the buds, which serve to trap insects. Therefore, as inferred, terpenes act as a protector against both high temperatures and insects too.

A description of the main terpenes in the cannabis plant and their medicinal use, are discussed on the following pages.

Myrcene

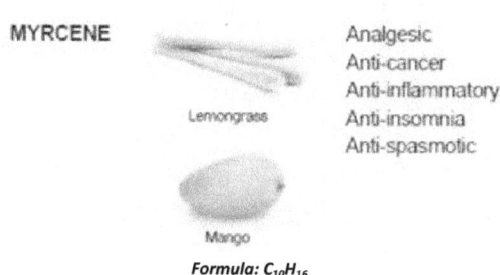

MYRCENE

Lemongrass

Mango

Analgesic
Anti-cancer
Anti-inflammatory
Anti-insomnia
Anti-spasmotic

Formula: $C_{10}H_{16}$
Boiling point: 167 C (333 F)

Myrcene, or β-myrcene, is a lineal (acyclic) *montoterpene* and besides cannabis, it is the main component of the essential oil of wild thyme, comprising 40% of its overall composition. It is also found at high concentrations plants such as hop, mango, sweet basil, lemongrass, verbena, and bay leaves.

The scent of myrcene is described as earthy, fruity, clove-like, and can be quite pungent in high doses.

Myrcene acts as an anti-inflammatory and is the sedative active ingredient found in hop. Myrcene is used in herbalism and in natural therapies to help with sleeping disorders.

Studies have shown myrcene to possess antimicrobial, antiseptic, antioxidant, and anti-carcinogen effects. In addition, myrcene has sedative, hypnotic, analgesic (pain relieving) and muscle relaxant properties. Studies also show that myrcene alters the blood-brain barrier, favoring the penetration of cannabinoids in the brain and increasing their effects. This means that this terpene enhances the beneficial effects of cannabinoids.

Myrcene is vital in the formation of other terpenes too and it synergizes their antibiotic effects.

Myrcene is the subject of a known rumor in that eating a ripe mango before indulging in cannabis medicine will increase the THC effects in the cannabis medicine. Mangos are known for their high myrcene content.

In a recent study, analyzing the composition of terpenes in indica varieties against sativa varieties revealed *a greater presence of myrcene in indica varieties by as much as 60%-80% of their composition.* A common belief is that indica varieties are more relaxing and sedative relative to sativa varieties. Although Myrcene is found in both strains of Cannabis, it is not found in hemp. It is hypothesized that Myrcene is responsible for the hypnotic effect in indica varieties, in addition to sedative and relaxing qualities.

Myrcene is the most prevalent terpene found in most varieties of cannabis and it is found in high amounts in lemongrass, mangos, hops, thyme, black pepper, and verbena. It is a known building block for menthol, citronella, and geraniol. Other scientific studies include analgesic, antibacterial, anti-cancer, anti-diabetic, anti-proliferative, anti-inflammatory, anti-insomnia and anti-spasmodic, anti-oxidant, antimicrobial, antiseptic, and muscle relaxing effects.

Beta-Caryophyllene (BCP)

β-CARYOPHYLLENE

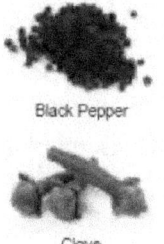

Black Pepper

Clove

Anti-bacterial
Anti-cancer
Anti-fungal
Anti-inflammatory
Anti-septic

Formula: $C_{15}H_{24}O$
Boiling point: 119 C (246 F)

Caryophyllene is an essential oil comprised of three compounds: alpha-caryophyllene (also known as humulene), beta-caryophyllene, and an oxidized caryophyllene (a result of the oxidation of both lemon balm and eucalyptus).

Beta-caryophyllene is a bicyclic **sesquiterpene** and, in addition to cannabis, is naturally found in basil, oregano, cinnamon bark, rosemary, hops , cloves, juniper, hyssop, yarrow, and black pepper and contributes to the latter's spiciness.

Therapeutic benefits include analgesic, anti-bacterial, anti-fungal, anti-inflammatory, bronchodilator and effective at reducing neuropathic pain. This terpene also has gastro-protective qualities and is good for gastrointestinal complications. BCP also binds to the CB2 receptor, in fact, it acts specifically on the body's CB2 cannabinoid pathways, and since CB2 is considered an endocannabinoid receptor (found in the body), BCP is being considered a cannabinoid. Since cannabinoids and terpenes are related, it should not come as much of a surprise to learn that terpenes can also trigger the body's endocannabinoid receptors.

The scent of *caryophyllene oxide* is what the sniffer drug dogs are trained to find.

Caryophyllene is less volatile than other terpenes and resists the process of decarboxylation, thus enabling its defectiveness in chromatography.

In the plant kingdom, *ß-caryophyllene* plays an important role in the protection of plants against insects and herbivores. *Caryophyllene oxide* increases the defense system of plants, functioning as an insecticide and an antifungal. It is very interesting to note that caryophyllene and the *CBC cannabinoid - cannabichromene* both join in the defense against fungi attacks. In addition, cannabis strains that contain both caryophyllene and cannabidiol (CBD) increase the anti-inflammatory and analgesic properties of the plant medicine.

Humulene

HUMULENE

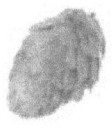

Hops

Anorectic
Anti-cancer
Anti-bacterial
Anti-inflammatory

Formula: $C_{15}H_{24}$
Boiling point: 198 C (388 F)

Humulene is commonly known as ***alpha-caryophyllene*** but is different in its mechanism of action relative to beta-caryophyllene.

A ***sesquiterpene***, humulene's scent has been described as robust, earthy, and herbaceous. Besides cannabis, Humulene is also found in pine trees, orange orchards, tobacco, sage, spearmint, ginger, Vietnamese coriander, hops basil, ginseng, and sunflowers. Humulene has anti-inflammatory effects and has the potential to be effective in managing autoimmune or inflammatory diseases. This terpene is also effective in treating conditions of edema and is anti-cancer. Humulene is similar to THCV because of its appetite suppressant activities.

Humulene is also commonly referred to as alpha-humulene or alpha-caryophyllene. Although humulene is related to beta-caryophyllene, it is a different isomer with different properties.

Therapeutic uses include *analgesic,* pain reliever; *antibacterial,* inhibits bacterial growth; *anti-inflammatory,* systemically reduces inflammation; *anti-proliferative,* inhibits cancer cell growth; *anorectic,* suppresses appetite and promotes weight loss.

Strains that include a noticeable high quantity of Humulene include Skunk, Swissmix from Switzerland and Bolivia's Amtbol 398

Pinene

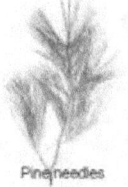

α-PINENE

Anti-bacterial
Anti-fungal
Anti-inflammatory
Bronchodilator

Pine needles

Formula $C_{10} H_{16}$
Boiling point: 155 C (311 F)

The familiar pine scent in cannabis is due to the Pinene terpene, includes both the alpha and beta isomer bicyclic monoterpenes, known as α-pinene (alpha), and β-pinene (beta), and is the main component of pine resin. This terpene is the most widely distributed terpene in nature. In fact, not only is it found in the plant kingdom, the two compounds are part of the chemical communication system of insects and even act as an insect repellent.

Alpha-pinene is the dominant of these two terpenes that is found in the cannabis plant.

In addition to cannabis, pinene is also found in the essential oils of many species of the fir trees especially pine. It is also found in medicinal herbs such as rosemary, basil, parsley, dill, peppermint, and the eucalyptus tree. Pinenes have significant antibiotic properties even against antibiotic resistant pathogens. Other therapeutic benefits include antiseptic; expectorant; bronchodilator and as such can be a treatment for asthma; it also increases mental focus and energy.

This compound has **significant** antibiotic properties, even against the strongest antibiotic resistant pathogens. The pinenes also possess significant anti-inflammatory properties, similar in action to myrcene. Pinene also acts as a bronchodilator in humans, when inhaled slowly. The addition of the pinenes in cannabis could allow a larger absorption of beneficial cannabinoids when smoking or vaporizing strains with a relatively high content of Pinene.

Alpha-pinene seems to be quite balanced within the various strains of cannabis with a usual quantity of 10% of the terpene group but not exceeding 15-20%.

Despite the above, this terpene was found at the highest level in the Sativa strain Super Silver Haze when analyzed by the Green House Seed Company. Other strains with a relative large amount of pinene include Jack Herer (Sativa), Chemdawg (Hybrid), Bubba Kush (Indica), and Trainwreck (Hybrid).

Limonene

LIMONENE 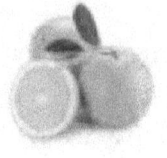 Anti-anxiety
Anti-bacterial
Anti-cancer
Anti-depressant
Anti-fungal
Bronchodilator

Citrus

Formula: C₁₀H₁₆
Boiling point: 176 C (349 F)

Limonene is a cyclic *monoterpene* and a main component of the essential oil of lemons and other citrus fruits and is where its name comes from. This terpene is the second most widely distributed terpene in nature and it is an intermediate product in other terpenes' biosynthesis. In contrast with pinene, limonene is not found in insects, yet it still has some repellent and insecticide effects. It is widely used in the food and pharmaceutical industries as flavoring. Recent research has been carried out to look at its usefulness in formulations of dermal patches, to improve the transdermal absorption of other active substances.

Studies on laboratory animals suggest that limonene has anxiolytic effects (inhibits anxiety), causing a rise of serotonin and dopamine neurotransmitters in the brain. Studies have shown that limonene in the environment, such as through aromatherapy, reduces depression in hospital patients. Limonene is also a strong immune stimulant and causes apoptosis or programmed cell death, in breast cancer cells.

Limonene is found in citrus fruit rinds, rosemary, and juniper. This terpene is often repulsive to predators and is a potent anti-fungal and anti-cancer agent. Other therapeutic benefits are anti-anxiety (anxiolytic), anti-bacterial, anti-cancer, anti-depressant, and bronchodilator and can dissolve gallstones. Limonene also enhances alertness and helps focus attention; it increases cerebral acetylcholine activity, which decreases memory loss. Limonene has been shown to both stimulate the immune system as well as be an effective cancer treatment.

This terpene is also commonly found in many strains of cannabis. Hybrid strains with high limonene terpenes include OG Kush, Super Lemon Haze, Jack the Ripper, and Lemon Skunk.

Linalool

LINALOOL

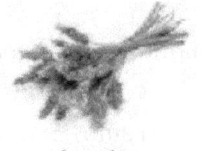

Lavender

Anti-anxiety
Anti-bacterial
Anti-convulsive
Anti-depressant
Anti-insomnia

Formula: $C_{10}H_{18}O$
Boiling Point: 198 C (388 F)

Linalool is a lineal *monoterpene* and is the main compound of the essential oil of lavender, but is also found in many other plants including cannabis.

The aroma of linalool is floral, similar to spring flowers with hints of citrus. Linalool is found in over 200 species of plants that are mainly from the families *Lamiaceae* (mints); *Lauraceae* (laurels, cinnamon, and rosewood) and *Rutaceae* (citrus fruits).

Therapeutic benefits of linalool include anti-stress, anti-bacterial, anti-convulsive, anti-depressant, anti-insomnia, anti-anxiety, and effective in pain management. It is found very useful as an anesthetic, anti-allergy, and a Broncho relaxant. Linalool is also used in the treatment of both psychosis and anxiety disorders plus it has been effectively used as an anti-epileptic agent (anti-seizure).

Linalool is also a very important precursor in the formation of Vitamin E.

Strains with a high Linalool content include LA Confidential (Indica), Lavender (Indica), Amnesia Haze (Sativa), and G-13 (Indica).

Eucalyptol also called Cineole

CINEOL

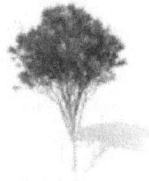

Tea Tree

Anti-bacterial
Anti-depressant
Anti-inflammatory
Anti-ischemic
Bronchodilator

Formula: $C_{10}H_{18}O$
Boiling point: 176 C (349 F)

Eucalyptol, also known as **Cineole**, is a *monoterpene* ester and is what makes up most of the essential oil of eucalyptus and is where it gets its name. The scent is described as spicy, refreshing, and minty and, in addition to cannabis, this terpene is found in rosemary, sage, bay leaves, wormwood, tea tree, mugwort, and eucalyptus.

Eucalyptol has been shown to assist with more conditions than most other terpenes, making it of great interest for research. This terpene can be applied topically to the skin and gums, or taken orally by being inhaled, drank as a tincture, or eaten. When taken orally or topically, it is important to dilute this essential oil.

Eucalyptol also acts as an insect repellent and insecticide, although it is produced by certain orchids to attract bees.

In a study comparing terpenes in Sativa and Indica varieties, it was found that eucalyptol, Carene, and Terpinolene are almost exclusively found in sativa varieties. Eucalyptol and Carene are found in proportions close to 5% and Terpinolene was found at proportions up to 20% of the total in sativa varieties while Indica varieties showed 1% or less.

The numerous health benefits of eucalyptus oil have attracted the attention of the entire world to explore its usage in aromatherapy as well as conventional medicine.

Therapeutic uses include analgesic, antibacterial, anti-fungal, anti-inflammatory, anti-proliferative (inhibits cancer cell growth) and antioxidant.

Eucalyptus essential oil is obtained from fresh leaves of the tall evergreen eucalyptus tree. The tree, which has the botanical name Eucalyptus Globules, is also known as fever tree, blue gum tree, or stringy bark tree. Eucalyptus is native to Australia and has spread in the past few centuries to other parts of the world including India, Europe, and South Africa. Though many countries produce eucalyptus oil in small quantities, the prime source of eucalyptus oil for the world is Australia.

Borneol

BORNEOL

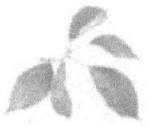

Camphor

Analgesic
Anti-insomnia
Anti-septic
Bronchodilator

Formula: $C_{10}H_{18}O$
Boiling point: 213 C (415 F)

Borneol is a bicyclic organic compound and a *monoterpene* that is easily oxidized to the ketone yielding camphor. It is also easily converted into menthol. Borneol is composed of two isoprene rings that are fused together making it larger than other monoterpenes found in cannabis such as limonene and smaller than sesquiterpenes such as beta-caryophyllene.

The scent can be described as menthol, pine, and woody. Borneol can also be found in cinnamon and wormwood, along with various strains of cannabis. Considered a calming sedative, its therapeutic benefits are analgesic, anti-insomnia, anti-septic and bronchodilator. It is also indicated for severe obstruction of the orifices, for heat syndromes, pain, and applied topically for a wide range of conditions. Borneol is a component of a number of essential oils and is a natural insect repellent. Borneol was also found to be an effective control mechanism to combat West Nile and other mosquito borne pathogens.

The therapeutic uses for borneol include *analgesic*, relieves pain; *antibacterial,* slows bacterial growth; *anti-fibrosis,* balances the body's fibrosis response to injury (controls scarring); *anti-fungal,* inhibits the growth of fungus; *anti-inflammatory,* systematically reduces the rate of inflammation; *antioxidant,* protects other molecules in the body from a loss of electrons.

Borneol is used in traditional Chinese medicine as 'moxa' and included in a very early Materia Medica that was written during the Ming Dynasty (1368-1644).

Terpinolene

TERPINOLENE

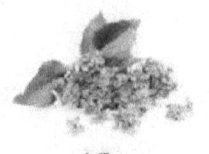

Lilac

Anti-bacterial
Anti-fungal
Anti-insomnia
Anti-septic

Formula: $C_{10}H_{16}$
Boiling point: 174 C (345 F)

Terpinolene, *a montoterpene*, is part of a group of terpenes from the group **terpinenes**. Terpinolene is also found in apples, cumin, coriander, lilac, marjoram, and tea tree. The scent is soft smoky or woody. Terpinolene has been used as an antiseptic for centuries. It also contains both anti-bacterial and anti-fungal properties. In addition, it is effective in treating insomnia as a blend of lilac and lavender.

Most cannabinoids and terpenes are either analgesic or anti-inflammatory, or both. However, terpinolene is neither BUT as with other cannabinoids, terpinolene fights cancer, is anti-fungal and antibacterial. It is also an effective sedative, which may be very beneficial to those in cancer treatment and have difficulty sleeping. When this terpene is combined with Cannabinol, the combination is a very effective and safe remedy for those having difficulty sleeping.

The therapeutic uses of terpinolene include *antibacterial,* slows bacterial growth; *antifungal* inhibits the growth of fungus; *anti-insomnia*, facilitates falling and staying asleep; *anti-prolific*, inhibits the growth of cancer cells; *antioxidant*, prevents damage to other molecules in the body from oxidization;

Tincture, Elixir, Syrup, Tisane, Infusion, Decoction

An herbal remedy is prepared to maintain health and/or to prevent, alleviate or cure a disease or ailment. In both Ayurvedic (traditional healing originating in India) and Traditional Chinese Medicine (TCM), tonics promote rejuvenation, regeneration and shining health.

An herb tonic must meet the following three conditions:

The herb must be non-toxic (no side effects or danger from long-term use exists);

The herb must promote wellness throughout the body and not limited to one system (ex. Circulatory, respiratory, etc.) **AND**

The herb must promote homeostasis in the body.

There is no question that cannabis meets the above definition of tonic.

Herbal preparations separate the soluble medicinal components of an herbal plant from its fibrous portion. Herbal preparations include *tinctures, elixir, syrup, tisanes (tea), decoctions, and infusions* defined as follows:

Tincture: an herbal extract using alcohol as the medium;

Elixir: an herbal extract using both alcohol and honey;

Syrup: a concentrated tea with the addition of honey, maple syrup or glycerin;

Tisane (tea): an herbal extract using water as the medium

Infusion: tea preparation using a "steeping" process;

Decoction: tea preparation using a "simmering" process

Decarbing Graph and Chart

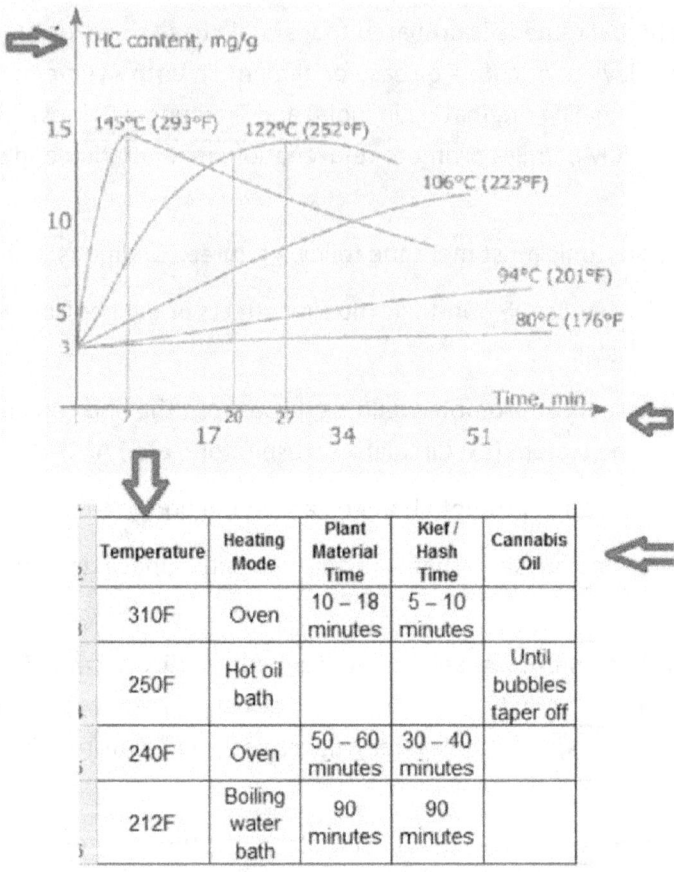

The first chart above refers to decarbing THCA to THC. At a temperature of 220-250 F, decarbing will convert THCA to THC in roughly 27 minutes when using about 15 grams of material. Extending the time up to 50 minutes may convert your THC to the degraded form of CBN.

The above graph and chart are for reference purposes only. Experimenting with the quantity, temperature and time can perfect a technique that works best for you and your condition.

Cannabis Infused Coconut Oil

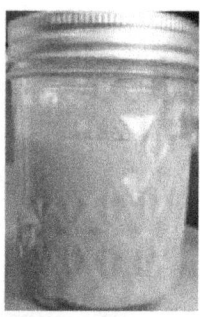

Infusing cannabis into oil is not new. The cannabinoids in cannabis are hydrophobic, meaning they are insoluble in water but soluble in lipids (oil/fat) and alcohol.

The healthiest oil to use for making cannabis infused oil is virgin coconut oil. Coconut oil has a number of health benefits on its own including high amounts of essential fatty acids (EFA) and beneficial saturated fats. Coconut oil contains a high amount of lauric acid, which is very beneficial for our immune system.

This recipe does not require that you decarb your cannabis in the oven first. Using the graph and chart on the previous page, turning THCA into THC occurs at a particular temperature for a specific duration of time. Heating beyond this point, results in your THC degrading to CBN.

Supplies required: (Substitute unsalted butter in place of coconut oil if desired by a ratio of 1-2 ounces of material to 1 pound of butter).

Cannabis material: trim/bud combination **or** a combination of various bud strains; the better the material, the better the oil will be; use 1.5-1.75 grams of bud material per ounce of coconut oil, which translates to ½ ounce of cannabis to 1 cup of organic virgin coconut oil;

Consider including your "spent" vaped cannabis material in this recipe too, as a way to maximize its use;

Extra virgin organic coconut oil: available in health food stores and most grocery stores

Grinder: a steel bud buster or coffee grinder

Scale: that measures in grams

Meat or candy thermometer: for testing temperature of heated oil

Crockpot

Timer:

Strainer/Cheesecloth/Coffee filter

Instructions:

First, measure your ingredients using the above ratio as an approximation;

Using a steel bud buster or clean coffee grinder, grind cannabis material to a "fine" consistency but not a fine powder;

Meanwhile, heat coconut oil in crockpot set to low. If using lecithin, add it to the oil at this point.

Once coconut oil reaches a temperature of 220 F – 250 F, stir in your ground cannabis material. Cover crockpot and set timer to 20 minutes. Do not remove the crockpot lid, as this will release the heat. (*Without the use of a thermometer, I followed the above method for 30 minutes; one tablespoon of infused oil in a cup of tea was enough to knock me out*).

Strain oil into a mason jar using a steel sieve lined with cheesecloth or a coffee filter; ensure to squeeze all oil out of the cannabis substance; save the remaining plant material to use as a poultice or topical compress, if desired, but store in your freezer until needed.

Coconut oil is an excellent choice in baking and can replace butter in most recipes. Use the cannabis infused oil in recipes for cookies or brownies; alternatively, add 1 teaspoon to a Chai Tea or other hot beverage for a quick and efficient medication.

Important Information:

Experiment with the amount and quality of plant material along with cooking time to determine what is best for you. Extending the cooking time and/or increasing the heat will increase the sedative effects of your medicine. Don't forget to *titrate* your medicine (start with a small amount and adjust upwards accordingly)

Soy Lecithin: Many advocate for the use of adding 1 teaspoon of soy lecithin to canna-oil/butter. The premise is that it increases the potency of the infusion. However, there is growing evidence that all soy products are GMO (genetically modified), despite any label to the contrary.

Tincture

EXTRACTUM CANNABIS

Extract of Cannabis

Ext. Cannab.—Extractum Cannabis indica P.I.

Prepare an extract by percolating 1000 Gm. of cannabis, in moderately coarse powder, using alcohol as the menstruum. Macerate the drug during forty-eight hours and then percolate it at a moderate rate until the drug is exhausted. Evaporate the percolate to a pilular consistence at a temperature not exceeding 70° C., and mix the mass thoroughly.

AVERAGE DOSE—Metric, 0.015 Gm.—Apothecaries, ¼ grain.

United States Pharmacopeia 1936 pg. 155

Cannabis oil, also known as concentrated cannabis extract, hash oil, weed oil, etc., is the traditional and historic form of cannabis medicine. Since the removal of cannabis from the US Pharmacopeia beginning with the 1942 edition, various solvents used to extract the cannabinoids from cannabis can be extremely dangerous.

If you are making your own oil, do NOT use Naphtha, butane, hexane nor Coleman fuel as your solvent because these are extremely dangerous to work with and can leave harmful residual impurities in the oil. To make cannabis oil, you need to use 99/100% Isopropyl alcohol or 190-proof grain alcohol (also known as Everclear).

Although there are a number of ways to make cannabis oil, the following method uses grain alcohol as the solvent and requires placing your high quality bud material in the freezer first in order that the trichomes stick to the bud rather than falling off during the grinding process.

The amount of cannabis bud and solvent to use is 1 lb. of high quality bud and 2 gallons of solvent. This will make approximately 60 grams of cannabis oil with amazing healing benefits to ingest over 90 days. One ounce of high quality buds and 500 ml of solvent will make approximately 3-5 grams of oil.

Materials required:

Cannabis buds: top quality with high THC content as well as high quantity of other cannabinoids

Solvent: ideally grain alcohol

Electric rice cooker

Electric candle warmer

Thermometer, fan, coffee filters

Stainless steel bowls, funnel/filter, mixing spoon

Oven mitts, safety gloves, safety glasses

Directions:

Step 1: Place the bone-dry cannabis buds in a container large enough to hold all the material

Step 2: First wash: add enough solvent to cover the cannabis and lightly crush the cannabis material for approximately three minutes. This first wash strips approximately 80% of the cannabinoids from the plant material into the solvent.

Step 3: Place a coffee-filter inside a funnel and filter the solvent from the cannabis material into another bowl or large bottle.

Step 4: Second wash: A second wash is required to remove the remaining 20% of cannabinoids from the plant material, therefore, repeat steps 2 and 3 by adding more solvent to the plant material and gently crush for another three minutes before filtering the solvent into the same container as your first wash.

Be extremely careful for the following steps:

In a well ventilated area with your safety glasses and the fan on:

Step 5: Pour the strained solvent into the rice cooker no more than ¾ full. Turn the rice cooker to high heat. As the solvent evaporates, continue adding more solvent into the rice cooker, not exceeding ¾ full, until all the solvent is in the rice cooker. Keep a good eye on the mixture as it cooks.

When there is approximately two inches of solvent left in the rice cooker, add a couple drops of water to boil off the last remaining amount of solvent. Put on your oven mitts, pick the unit up and gently swirl the contents in the rice cooker to aid in evaporating the solvent. The addition of the water will cause the oil to bubble, crackle and possibly smoke. This is completely normal.

Step 6: Gently pour the oil into a stainless steel or glass container. Place the container on a candle/coffee warmer.

Cannabinoid Patents

With the adoption of the **UN's Single Convention on Narcotic Drugs**, the control of cannabis production, cultivation, and distribution is restricted except under license.

In the UK, the *UK Home Office* licensed GW Pharma Limited to grow cannabis for research purposes.

In the US, the NIH and NIDA have contracted with the University of Mississippi to grow research grade cannabis.

The purported lack of research has certainly **not** stopped the prolific amount of patent applications filed by these authorized government authorized organizations from recognizing and capitalizing on the wide range of medical uses.

Since the adoption of the International Treaty to control cannabis production, cultivation and distribution, both GW Pharma and the USA have continuously filed patent applications on the medicinal benefits of cannabis. Examples of some of the patents for inventions on using specific cannabinoids for specific purposes are included on the following pages.

THCV to Treat Diabetes and Pre-diabetes

Patent number: WO2013076471 A1

Publication date: May 30, 2013

Applicant: GW Pharma Limited

Abstract: The present invention relates to the phytocannabinoids Tetrahydrocannabivarin (THCV) for use in the protection of pancreatic islet cells. Preferably, the pancreatic islet cells to be protected are beta cells. More preferably, the protection of the pancreatic islet cells maintains insulin production at levels, which are able to substantially control or improve control of blood glucose levels in a patient.

THCV and CBDV for Brain Cancer

Phytocannabinoids for use in the treatment of cancer

Application number: US 13/634,343

Application number: 14/343,877

Date: PCT filed Sep 10, 2012

Date per ss371 (c) (1), (2), (4) date Mar 10, 2014

Assignees: GW Pharma

Abstract: The present invention relates to the use of phytocannabinoids in the treatment of cancer. More particularly, it relates to the use of phytocannabinoids in the treatment of tumor cell invasion and cell migration or metastases. Cancers where invasion and cell migration plays a key role in prognosis include brain tumors, more particularly gliomas, and most particularly Glioblastoma multiform (GBM) and breast cancers. The phytocannabinoids Tetrahydrocannabivarin (**THCV**) and Cannabidivarin (**CBDV**) alone or in combination with each other and/or other phytocannabinoids, particularly *CBD, THC, and CBG or their respective acids* are of particular use.

Intestinal Inflammatory Diseases

Publication number: US 2014/0343136 A1

Publication date: Nov 20, 2014

Applicant: GW Pharma Limited, Salisbury (GB)

Abstract: The present invention relates to one or more of the phytocannabinoids THCV, CBG, CBC, and CBDV for use in the treatment of intestinal inflammatory diseases. Preferably, the intestinal inflammatory disease is *either ulcerative colitis or Crohn's disease*.

CBG for Alzheimer's

Cannabinoids for use in the treatment of Neurodegenerative diseases or Disorders

Application number: 14/128,208

PCT filed Jun 29, 2012

Assignee: GW Pharma

Abstract: The present invention relates to CBG for use in the prevention or treatment of neurodegenerative diseases or disorders. Preferable the cannabinoids are CBC, CBDV, and or CBDVA. More preferable the neurodegenerative disease or disorder to be prevented or treated is Alzheimer's disease.

CBG for Mood Disorders

Application number: 13/869,247

Date: Apr 24, 2013

Assignee: GW Pharma Limited

Abstract: The present invention relates to the use of CBG type compounds and derivatives thereof in the treatment of mood disorders.

Closing Remarks

The intention of this book is to emphasize the historical medicinal use of cannabis, despite the current muscled fight for control of this plant.

Due to the mass hybridization in cannabis strains over the past several decades, the distinction between Sativa and Indica has blurred. As breeders strived to produce strains with higher potency, larger yields, and shorter flowering times, a number of strains have very similar cannabinoid profiles. As a result, the terpenes in cannabis play a more important role than ever before in terms of selecting a particular strain for your specific purpose. As patients become better educated on cannabis medicine, they will then become discerning consumers dictating better quality product and professional information.

Since the discovery of the cannabinoid receptors (CB1 and CB2) along with the endogenous cannabinoids anandamide and 2-AG in the 1990's, scientists continue to study this area to gain a better understanding of the key physiological functions of our endocannabinoid system.

In modern Western society, we have come to accept that "traditional" medicine is the same as "mainstream" or "allopathic" medicine, which is synthetic pharmaceutical medicine.

Imagine what our planet and life would be like if the medicinal and industrial use of the cannabis plant was not ostracized in favor of private corporate greed.

Definitions

Analog: one of a group of chemical compounds similar in structure but different in respect to elemental composition

Auto-Flowering: flowering based on age rather than light cycle

Biological activity: In pharmacology, describes the beneficial or adverse effects of a drug on living matter.

Bract: A leaf stipule that is located on both sides of the axis of the petiole or leaf stalk (underneath part of a bud); describes leaf structure

Calyx: five-part carpel structure of the staminate flower or the five part fused tubular sheath that surrounds the ovule and pistils; describes floral structure; contain high concentrations of trichomes, or glands that secrete THC and other cannabinoids and terpenes

Chemistry: the science that deals with the composition and properties of substances along with various elementary forms of matter

Chemotaxonomy: the identification and classification of organisms by comparative analysis of their biochemical composition

Cola: also known as the terminal bud; the main cola forms at the very top of the plant and is sometimes referred to as the apical bud; refers to the "bud site" where tight female flowers bloom; see also inflorescence

Decarboxylation: a chemical reaction that removes a carboxyl group from an organic compound; in cannabis, raw cannabinoids are decarbed with heat converting, for example, CBGA into CBG (also called decarbing)

Elucidate to make clear; to provide clarification; to explain

Glandular trichomes: secretory or resin glands where cannabinoids accumulate (see trichomes below)

Hermaphrodites: a plant containing both male and female reproduction organs; natural hermaphrodites with are usually sterile, but artificially induced hermaphrodites (known as feminized seeds), are treated with silver thiosulfate

Homologous: having the same alleles or genes in the same order of arrangement; of the same chemical type, but differing by a fixed increment of an atom or a constant group of atoms

Inflorescence: the "bud site" the cluster of flowers arranged on a stem composed of a main branch or a complicated arrangement of branches, also referred to as *cola*

Medicalization: the process by which all human conditions and problems come to be defined and treated as 'medical conditions', and thus, the subject of "medical study, diagnosis, prevention, and treatment"

Metabolism: any basic process of organic functioning or operating; the sum of the physical and chemical processes in an organism by which its material substance is produced, maintained, and destroyed, and by which energy is made available

Pharmacological activity: This is the same as biological activity above.

Pharmacology: the science dealing with the preparation, uses, and especially the effects of drugs

Phenotype: observable characteristics or traits including size, shape, color, aroma, bud density, flavor, etc.

Pistils: The red or white hairs that grow out of the bud; their purpose is to collect pollen from the males; begin as white and progressively darken over the course of the plants maturation; contribute little to potency and taste but important none the less in development

Stipule: leaf spur

Trichomes: Also known as, *glandular trich*omes or "crystals"; when magnified appear hair like; trichomes are described as translucent, mushroom-shaped glands seen on the surface of the cannabis bud; clear bulbous globes that produce aromatic oils (terpenes) and cannabinoids; originally developed by plant as a protective defense mechanism; they secrete resin (known as 'kief 'when dry)

Trichrome: trichrome – with the extra 'r' is defined as having the ability to see three colors"

Sources Used

http://norml.org/library/item/introduction-to-the-endocannabinoid-system

http://www.ncbi.nlm.nih.gov/pmc/articles/PMC20983/

R Adams with S Loewe, Charles Jelinek and Hans Wolff, Tetrahydrocannabinol homologs with marihuana activity, IX, JACS 1941:63:1971-3.

R Adams with CM Smith and S Loewe, Tetrahydrocannabinol homologs and analogs with marihuana activity, X, JACS 1941:63:1973-6.

R Adams with CK Cain and S Loewe, Tetrahydrocannabinol analogs with marihuana activity, XI, JACS 1941:63:1977-8.

R Adams with CK Cain, WD McPhee and RB Wearn, Structure of cannabidiol, XII, Isomerization to tetrahydrocannabinols, JACS 1941:63:2209-13.

http://www.leafscience.com/2013/09/21/5-health-benefits-of-cannabichromene-cbc/

http://www.google.com/patents/US20140343136

http://stks.freshpatents.com/Gw-Pharma-Limited-nm1.php

http://www.naturalnews.com/022630_soy_food_phytic_acid.html

http://www.cureyourowncancer.org/

http://www.cureyourowncancer.org/1974-study-showing-cannabis-kills-cancer-cells-antineoplastic-activity-of-cannabinoids.html

http://www.ncbi.nlm.nih.gov/pubmed/21182490

https://www.projectcbd.org/condition/29/Liver-Disease

http://www.wjgnet.com/1007-9327/full/v14/i40/6109.htm#__sec4

http://www.fundacion-canna.es/en/terpenes

http://www.thelibertybeacon.com/2013/08/30/monsanto-gmos-big-pharma-and-the-government-theyre-killing-us-11650/

About the Author

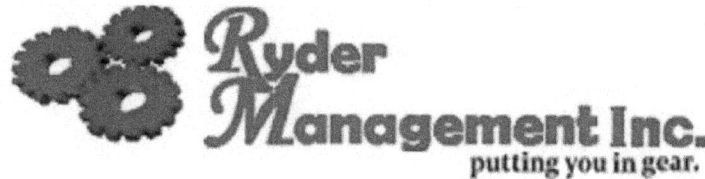

Located in London, Canada, *Ryder Management Inc* is a publisher whose primary focus is on natural healing remedies. Rydermgt acts as an umbrella organization for a number of independent authors with common and like goals of helping others achieve optimal health naturally.

If you enjoyed this book, please tell others; otherwise please tell us!

Other Kindle books written by Ryder Management Inc can be viewed at our author page at the following Amazon link: http://www.amazon.com/Ryder-Management-Inc./e/B00ICGMCRS

Please let us know your thoughts at the following email link: info@Rydermanagement.ca